Energy

Learning Reiki Symbols and Master Chakra Usage

(Learn How to Cleanse Your Aura, Eliminate Depression, Increase Positive Energy and Improve Health With Reiki Treatment and Meditation)

William Mitchell

Published by Rob Miles

William Mitchell

All Rights Reserved

Energy: Learning Reiki Symbols and Master Chakra Usage (Learn How to Cleanse Your Aura, Eliminate Depression, Increase Positive Energy and Improve Health With Reiki Treatment and Meditation)

ISBN 978-1-989990-35-3

All rights reserved. No part of this guide may be reproduced in any form without permission in writing from the publisher except in the case of brief quotations embodied in critical articles or reviews.

Legal & Disclaimer

The information contained in this book is not designed to replace or take the place of any form of medicine or professional medical advice. The information in this book has been provided for educational and entertainment purposes only.

The information contained in this book has been compiled from sources deemed reliable, and it is accurate to the best of the Author's knowledge; however, the Author cannot guarantee its accuracy and validity and cannot be held liable for any errors or omissions. Changes are periodically made to this book. You must consult your doctor or get professional medical advice before using any of the suggested remedies, techniques, or information in this book.

Upon using the information contained in this book, you agree to hold harmless the Author from and against any damages, costs, and expenses, including any legal fees potentially resulting from the application of any of the information provided by this guide. This disclaimer applies to any damages or injury caused by the use and application, whether directly or indirectly, of any advice or information presented, whether for breach of contract, tort, negligence, personal injury, criminal intent, or under any other cause of action.

You agree to accept all risks of using the information presented inside this book. You need to consult a professional medical practitioner in order to ensure you are both able and healthy enough to participate in this program.

TABLE OF CONTENTS

INTRODUCTION 1

CHAPTER 1: WELCOME TO REIKI 4

CHAPTER 2: STRESS FROM YOUR DAILY ACTIVITIES 12

CHAPTER 3: REIKI BASICS 24

CHAPTER 4: REIKI INITIATION 38

CHAPTER 5: THE RELIGIOUS MYTHS CONTINUE 47

CHAPTER 6: THE REIKI IDEALS 58

CHAPTER 7: THE PRINCIPLES AND PILLARS OF REIKI 73

CHAPTER 8: PRACTICING REIKI 87

CHAPTER 9: THE REIKI HEALING TOOL 95

CHAPTER 10: OTHER REIKI USES 100

CHAPTER 11: HOW TO START HELPING OTHERS 107

CHAPTER 12: UNDERSTANDING AURAS AND HOW THEY ARE AFFECTED BY REIKI 112

CHAPTER 13: ATTRIBUTES OF A REIKI MASTER 125

CHAPTER 14: REIKI AND MEDITATION 128

CHAPTER 15: THE THIRD EYE AND REIKI 132

CHAPTER 16: WHAT IS COMMUNITY-BASED REIKI? 136

CHAPTER 17: MY INTRODUCTION TO REIKI 146

CHAPTER 18: ANGELIC REIKI BASICS SYNOPSIS 153

CHAPTER 19: A TYPICAL USUI REIKI SESSION 157

CHAPTER 20: ABOUT CHAKRAS INCLUDING THE THIRD EYE 160

CHAPTER 21: CRYSTAL CLEANSING TECHNIQUES 173

CHAPTER 22: PHYSICAL HEALING 188

CONCLUSION 202

Introduction

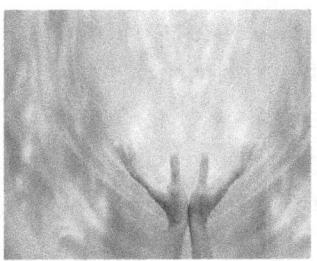

In this day and age, we are all forced to work hard and run around to get things done. We no longer live in a world where we can exist at our own pace, and it does not look to improve anytime soon. That being the case, we need to find ways to slow down and realign ourselves with our inner purpose, so that we may live the best life possible. As we learn to live up to the purpose of our inner selves, we find that things fit into place, and energy flows much easier, making daily and long term goals much easier to meet.

The following chapters will discuss some of the ways to practice energy healing, and how it will positively affect your life. The subject of energy healing is very broad, but it is deeply rooted in Eastern culture. Recently, these practices have made their way into the Western world and can act in tandem with traditional Western medicine to cure what ails us.

There are many ways to improve our lives through energy healing, and this book will discuss the basis of these practices, and go more in depth with the concepts of meditation, Reiki, guided imagery and much more.

You will discover how important it is to align your daily life with your inner purpose and your spiritual well-being. Even if you can't change your job or circumstances, there are little things we can do every single day to become more aligned with our true self, and the more we tap into that, the better off we will be.

Here, you will also find guided meditation sessions to help you on your way to practicing energy healing every day.

There are plenty of books on this subject on the market, thanks again for choosing this one! Every effort was made to ensure it is full of as much useful information as possible. Please enjoy!

Chapter 1: Welcome To Reiki

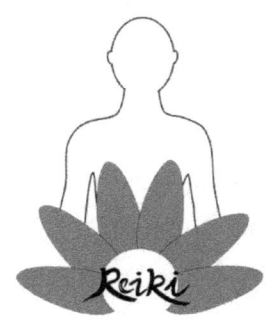

What Is Reiki?
Reiki is a Japanese word meaning universal life energy. At present, that word is being used to identify the Usui Natural Healing System (Usui Shiki Ryoho), a name given in homage to its discoverer, Mikao Usui. Laugh means universal and refers to the spiritual part, to the energetic essence cosmic, which interpenetrates all things and surrounds all places.
Ki is the individual life energy that surrounds our bodies, keeping them alive, and is present, flowing, in all living

organisms. When Ki energy leaves a body, that body ceases to have life. Reiki is a process of meeting these two energies: the universal energy with our physical portion, and occurs after the person is subjected to a process of tuning or initiation into the method, done by a trained teacher.

Reiki is an energy similar to radio waves and can be applied effectively, both locally and remotely. It is not like electricity, it does not produce short circuits, and it does not destroy nerves or the most fragile tissues. It is harmless energy, without side effects, without contraindications, compatible with any type of therapy or treatment. It is practical, safe, and efficient, and, by means of technique, it balances the seven chakras or centers of the subtle force of energy located between the base of the column and the top of the head.

When we use Reiki energy, we are applying light-energy, trying to recover and maintain physical, mental, emotional, and spiritual health. It is a natural method of balancing, restoring, perfecting, and healing the bodies, creating a state of harmony to the being.

Reiki Advantages and Benefits

Reiki is similar to a radio wave and can be applied properly in the same place or at a distance. It is above time and space, thus allowing reprogramming past events and coordinating future events. Energy is not manipulative. The practitioner simply places his hands, and the energy flows in the intensity and quality determined by the recipient.

It is not necessary to undress the patient during the application, as energy penetrates through anything. The therapist does not need to know the diagnosis of the pathology to successfully carry out the treatment. Reiki energizes and does not wear out the practitioner because the technique does not use the "Chi" or "Ki" of the practitioner, but the Vital Energy of the Universe.

Reiki is an optimal resource to balance the seven main chakras, which are located from the base of the column to the top of the head. Reiki quickly relieves physical pain.

Consider the person holistically, in the physical, emotional, mental, and spiritual bodies, not only taking into account the suppression of the pathology but returning it to a natural and desirable state of well-being and happiness. The Reiki practice is incorporated into the context of alternative therapeutic practices recognized by the World Health Organization (WHO). It can be used both in the treatment of oneself and in the treatment of other people, plants, and animals.

How Reiki Works

Western culture is based on a Newtonian-Cartesian conception, which is committed to the study of the parts to reach the whole. This view is widely questioned today. Quantum physics itself, through research on the atom and nuclear energy, shows that, at the smallest level, matter is at the same time energy.

Modern scientists have analyzed the world with an incredible degree of sophistication. The material world is divided into smaller and smaller particles, and, in the end, what we find are waves of energy (quanta). We discover the simple truth that energy precedes matter, just as emotions and thoughts precede action.

That vision of the world, new in the West, very ancient in the East, proposes that all that exists is energy. Energy is the basic reality that condenses, balances, and forms matter. With the modern formula of Albert Einstein ($E = mc^2$), it was scientifically proven that matter and energy are convertible and interchangeable. For example, the elements enriched in plutonium and uranium can be transformed into pure energy (explosions), as what happened in Hiroshima and Nagasaki, and also that energy can be transformed into matter since they are dimensions of the same reality.

From the time of Chinese, Tibetan, and Indian medicines, and even from the time of medieval alchemists, there are millenary techniques that teach us that matter, in fact, is transformed and can be molded with the intervention of greater energy.

Energy is energy; there is no bad energy. There is only good or poorly directed energy. In a healthy person, energy flows freely through our physical body, flowing through "paths" or chakras, energy meridians, and nadis. It also surrounds the energy field, which we call the aura. That energy force nourishes our organs and cells and regulates vital functions. When that energy is blocked, and the circulation of that energy is interrupted, a dysfunction occurs in the organs and tissues of our body.

By virtue of physical, emotional, mental, and spiritual excesses, we release energies, and these releases generate "energy knots" or "energy blocks" that interrupt or impede the normal flow of vital energy, causing dysfunction in the organs and tissues of the body, which, consequently, causes the disease due to poor functioning or malfunction of the organs and glands.

The Reiki technique uses total energy, from which the entire universe is constituted. It is the original energy of everything and of all beings that we capture and channel after the initiation (tuning) and activation of the energy centers (chakras). After being tuned in, we become channels of this cosmic energy, being able to direct it by placing our hands on the affected area. The hands emit vibrations that dissolve harmful nodes. In this way, we come to intervene effectively in matter, in other energy fields and in consciousness, which leads to a natural state of well-being, fullness, harmony, and balance.

Reiki heals by passing through the affected part of our energy field, raising the vibratory level inside and outside our physical body, where feelings and thoughts are lodged in the form of energy nodules, which act as barriers to our normal flow of energy vital. There are many who live with these barriers throughout a lifetime, minimizing their quality of life.

In a Reiki session, the amount of energy received by the patient is determined by the patient himself since the Reikian therapist is limited to directing the energy, and the provider (the Cosmos) delivers it unlimitedly.

Chapter 2: Stress From Your Daily Activities

Stress could have had an impact on your health, but maybe you don't realize that, thinking sickness is causing the annoying headache, repetitive insomnia or decreasing work efficiency in your workplace.

Stress usually affect your appearance body, your thoughts, your feelings, and your behavior. Knowing and recognizing common stress symptoms can help you manage them. However there's not much effective treatment of stress, only few ones are actually truly effective. Stress left unnoticed over time will lead to health issues, such as drained energy, diabetes, high blood pressure, obesity, heart disease, etc.

Stress drain energy

Human body isn't built suitable or compatible with extended experience of physical, mental or emotional stress over time without facing terrible repercussions. If it becomes deeply overworked continual fatigue would result. It might seem normal as the weakness isn't much or obvious yet. But when unchecked and prolonged can dramatically reduce the exact nutrients you need to create energy such as the B vitamins and magnesium, most paramount if dietary intake is low.

Anxiety, which can be accompanied by stress, can also help to over-stigate the stress response and to increase nutrient depletion.

Roots Of The Problem Need Concentration

It was opined by Elizabeth Scott (2018) that they always try to remove the underlying cause whenever someone tries to heal because that's what they believe to be a disorder. However, if you remove only the obvious sign, there would still be the core of the problem left. On the physical body, the indicator manifested itself to pull that root to your notice. Instead of noticing it and seeing what should be done about it, the root will take effect in your system much more drastically if you only take care of the obvious sign. It is feasible to develop what was there as asthma could become an enormous disaster for one's life. If the root would be removed, it cannot simply be removed and dissolved just like that. It's got to be removed and worked out somehow. These healing attempts are a very juvenile process, it's a very infantile thing to do.

Quite a lot of Individuals haven't yet understood and experienced life in any good depth; they

have only seen life in the physical dimension, so they think that the biggest thing they can do is to soothe an individual from his physical pain at that time. It shouldn't have been so.

We are pulled the same time in many directions of today's busy globe. At home and at work, we have duties, and sometimes it all gets too much. Our bodies are beginning to let us know we feel the stress of our everyday lives. Stress feelings are triggered by the instinct of our body to protect itself. During emergencies such as when you need to get out of a speeding car, this natural reaction is nice. But stress can trigger side effects that are unhealthy if it is not correctly managed.

Your spirit soul and the physical body is running extra time as it deals with each day challenge. You're simply not equipped to cope with all the greater strength. You can start to sense aggravating, afraid, worried, and uptight. Which can lead to severe health problems such as high blood pressure, heart illness, and diabetes if your stress is not kept under control.

You're late for work, the children won't stop yelling, your boss hunted you because you turned in a report late, your neighbor's dog won't stop barking, you owe tax thousands of dollars that you don't even have. You're under severe stress. At times, it serves a beneficial reason, because the pressure is clearly a normal part of lifestyles.

Stress can encourage you to get that advertising at work or run the final mile in a marathon race. If you don't get proper check on your stress and you allow it to become lengthy-term, it could critically intrude deep into your job, the circle of relatives existence, and health. Greater than half of Americans say they combat merely with friends and loved ones because of pressure, and a little more than 70% say they witnessed real body and emotional signs of mental or emotional strain-out, this stress is affecting their health.

Stress Sources

Everybody has distinct causes of strain. In line with studies, work stress is top of the listing. Forty percent of U.S. employees confess to office stress, and one-quarter say that paintings are their existence's greatest motive of stress.

Divorce
Getting married
Lengthy working hours
Dismissal at workplace
Packing load to a new home
Chronic illness or injury
A loved one's loss of life
Be dissatisfied at work
inflation of financial duties

Working in any harmful environment
Had to give a lecture before a co-worker
Looking after an old or sick member of the family
Having an exorbitant or massive workload
Be worried about your likelihood of success or risk of dismissal
Hostility or discrimination at work, particularly if your business organization isn't always supportive
Deficient leadership, uncertain expectations of your activity or having no say in choice-making
The Stresses On Life Can Also Have Some Drastic Effect:
Mental disturbances (instability, anxiety, sorrow, feelings of shame, low self-assurance or disgust).
Horrifying occurrences such as extreme weather events, robbery, or violence against you or your loved ones.
Sometimes the stress comes from within, not from outside. Just worrying about a lot of things, you can pressure yourself out.
Most of these can bring pressure to spirit, soul, and body:

Fear and uncertainty. When you hear on the news frequently about the risk of attacks around the world, widespread global-warming, and contaminants, it can make you feel stressed, particularly as you feel that you have no control over these happenings. Although crises are invariably very rare occurrences, their lively media coverage may make them appear to be more probable than they really are to happen. Fears can end up coming nearer as well, Along with constantly thinking that you're not going to complete a project at work or that you won't have enough income to pay for your tax and expenses.

Opinions and mentalities. How you view the world or a specific circumstance can determine if it causes stress. If your TV set is robbed and you take the stance, for instance, you say "That's ok, my insurance company's going to provide a replacement" you're going to be less stressed than if you believe, "My TV's gone and I'm never going to recover it! In fact, what if they return to my home to rob again?" "Similarly, individuals who feel like doing a great job at work will be less stressed by a large upcoming project than individuals who are worried that they are incredibly not prepared nor up to the task.

Expectations that are unrealistic. Nobody is really perfect. Expectation to do everything right all the time leads to stress, when they do not happen as expected.

Adjustments can happen in our lives. Any significant shift in life can be stressful-even a happy occurrence such as a wedding or job promotion. More unpleasant occurrences can be important sources of stress, such as divorce, major economic setback, or death of a relative.

Depending on your character and how you react to circumstances, your stress level will vary. Some individuals let themselves bounce off everything. Work stresses and stressors in life are only minor bumps on the highway for them. Others are simply worried about getting ill.

Preventing Stress

Stress in varying degrees is part of our lives; some of it can be known in advance and minimized, while some of it takes us by surprise and is inevitable, and some of the stress we face is predictable and chronic, but are not totally avoidable. The best we can do is handle the pressure we face by finding various methods to alleviate it. A "patterned" solution to stress management is best — one involving approaches that minimize stress where necessary, Other strategies that help us think less stressful about things when we can't prevent them, and extra resilience- building strategies that allow us to deal more efficiently with whatever happens. Most of us, however, understandably want a ' magic bullet ' of stress relief — one thing we can do every day to alleviate the daily grind stress. And having one daily stress relief habit will create a substantial difference in the stress level we feel. The catch? That one thing for everyone can be distinct.

While daily stress relievers are not one-size-fits-all, there are a few stress relievers' categories that work particularly well for many individuals:

Meditation
Meditation can be discovered as a good and even spiritual practice and can come in different forms in nearly all cultures. Whether for a few minutes or a long period, by being consistent and making it a regular exercise, you reap a broad variety of advantages. And while a brief session can still bring advantages, it can create resilience in long-term practice. Here's more about the advantages of meditation and various meditation kinds.

Exercise
For optimal health and the prevention of circumstances such as cancer and obesity, health scientists suggest a daily dose of exercise, and exercise is also a good reliever of stress. There are health advantages on many fronts for those who go to spin school, walk the dog in the morning, or find other methods to work physical exercise into their day. But you may not understand that exercise while improving longevity and quality of life, increases resilience to stress. It is one of the most difficult relievers of stress to

start and hang on to, but also one of the most fulfilling.

Here's how to get your exercise routine launched.

Do those things that put you in a good mood

Focus more on the positive aspect – being in a good mood – indicates that when individuals do tiny stuff that increases their mood, it produces an ' upswing path ' of positive emotions that merely leads to enhanced resilience to stress. (The more complex explanation is that they will increase your understanding of your possibilities, your enhanced mood will give you more

incentive to take advantage of these possibilities, yet this urge to establish resources leads to more beneficial moods; it's a self-perpetuating cycle.) So doing one little thing every day can generate something much bigger that enables you to overcome stress and at the same time maintain a smile on your face.

The right time to seek help

Here is just a list of symptoms when you feel stressed that you may encounter. Visit health practitioner if you did attempt the tips above and believe you still need assistance in handling your stress as expressed by American Family Physicians Academy in 2016.

Chapter 3: Reiki Basics

The foundation of the term Reiki is from 2 Japanese words, Rei meaning God's Wisdom or maybe Higher Ki and Power which means life force energy.

The Japanese healing and stress-reduction therapy literally means spiritually guided life force energy.

Reiki is dependant on the concept that health is out of the Ki streaming through as well as close to an individual, instead of the problem of the actual physical body. Ki is the explanation of why the actual physical organs feature in a healthful manner, when the flow in case Ki is blocked and disrupted, it negatively impacts the entire body, leading to the illness.

Ki responds to an individual's feelings and thoughts, therefore good feelings assist the Ki flow much more easily through the body to help enhanced health. Negative feelings contribute to a bad flow of Ki to add to reduced vitality and health. Even

Western medicine is beginning to recognize the mind body connection as well as the ability to improve/worsen health issues. To know how the mind body connection works, you have to comprehend which all of the organs are linked to the central nervous system through the nerves which transmit communications back and forth from the human brain, consequently the mind of ours is much more than the mind itself.

Reiki (pronounced ray key) is a kind of healing, in which a healer lays the hands of her on the components of the Japanese-reiki-healing body which will be in pain or call for healing. Energy (ki) is through the healer's hands to the components of the body that lack electricity. For Western reiki, you will find fixed hand positions, typically beginning with the head and then shifting down to the foot. With Japanese reiki, the therapy is provided exclusively centered on the location in which there's discomfort or pain. For instance, people usually carry a great deal of stress in the shoulders of theirs and lower back, therefore the healing can start the place that the person carries probably the most stress. In case you do not have some specific pain and also simply wish to have rest, then the session is able to begin from the head and walk right down to the foot.

Reiki gives restoration and relaxation of health. Additionally, it functions to prevent illnesses and also keeps you healthy. In case you're feeling tired, mentally or physically, it works as a good option for a massage. In several instances, it is able to assist the healing process after an operation and relieve pain. You will find hospices in North America that provide reiki to the patients of theirs to relieve some pain and enable them to relax.

Lots of people confuse the Japanese tradition of Reiki with massage or meditation, though it is really a totally distinct exercise with origins greatly embedded in Japanese tradition and spiritualism. If you have never ever experienced Reiki, it may help understanding its purpose and origins.

Many people credit Hawayo Takata, a Japanese female, with Reiki's roots and the spread of its on the West in the late twentieth century. Nevertheless, the International Center for Reiki Training founder William Rand has conducted research that is significant and also found references to Reiki dating to the mid 1800s. Takata's effort to distribute Reiki around the world remains crucial to the practice 's history. She produced tapes and also wrote newspapers to describe Reiki's benefits and purpose.

For a few years, Reiki remained confined to Japan. Nevertheless, it spread on the West as Reiki masters started offering classes & workshops created to instruct the craft. Interest increased in the United States, Europe, along with various other regions of the planet. It today serves as probably the most popular way of stress relief as well as energy influence for human beings.

Reiki can serve as a means to adjust as well as steer the body 's energy. Practitioners attempt to cleanse other issues and energy blockages which stall healing and prevent restoration. For example, Reiki is commonly utilized to assist sufferers of chronic pain and disease. While Reiki does not cure the illness or get rid of the injury, it can help the body produce the perfect environment for healing.

All healing starts with self healing. Reiki healing starts with the Reiki practitioner with a Reiki job, placing the hands of theirs on the individual to be healed, without stress. The life force energy referred to as Ki is the thing that creates the healing moving throughout the Chakras in the facilities of the tips and the palms of every finger. Reiki may additionally be delivered as distance healing, not simply to people, but additionally to cats, dogs, along with various other creatures. Numerous creatures readily recognize the Reiki energy. Occasionally they are going to reject the Reiki energy in case they're passing over, and in case the Reiki healing is not sufficient, it'll make the passing with no pain.

Reiki power requires no direction; the professional will be informed when you should replace the job. At times the Reiki healer is going to guide the receiver by way of a visualization procedure, and describe what is going on throughout the consultation. A session is able to keep going more than an hour and continues so long as the power sensations continue. Whenever a Reiki healer starts the therapeutic session, he or maybe she can't guarantee which the receiver is going to be healed. The Reiki energy appears to have ahead of its to promote, going to the place that the problem is and not always the place that the real pain is felt.

What exactly are the advantages of Reiki?

Reiki's main function lies in stress reduction. It soothes the brain and body by siphoning electricity in good directions and removing blockages that promote stress. Numerous individuals additionally experience pain relief, symptom minimization from illnesses, and also improved rest. It can likewise hasten recovery from surgery along with other medical procedures. Other healing techniques and reiki function as companions to modern day medicine and not as substitutes for them.

The Reiki Principles

Another advantage to Reiki is the fact that by living by the Reiki concepts, you are able to construct very good karma which will provide you much more positivity. Here are a few affirmations that are fundamental to the Reiki strategy.

Simply for today, I won't be angry It is a reminder of ours to let go of the anger of ours so we might have peace of mind. Additionally, anger is a bad emotion that causes energy blockages in the energy field of ours. Reiki is ideal for eliminating these energy blockages which could later affect us on an actual level. Therefore for today, allow it to go so the energy of yours can flow freely.

Simply for these days, I won't worry is additionally another negative emotion to give off. Whenever we stress about issues or situations we're placing that bad energy out into the universe. We're continuously asking The Universe Just how can I perform you? What we do not recognize is the Universe is replying with Now, just how can I serve you? We do get what we place into the Universe, therefore for today we need to keep it positive!

Simply for these days, I am going to be grateful From probably the deepest part of the heart of yours (intention is) that is important, be grateful for all you've in life. Friends, home life, a stable home, a loving pet, a good job, whatever it might be, be thankful it's there for you.

Simply for these days, I am going to do the work of mine really Put forth the best effort of yours with admiration for yourself and others.

Simply for these days, I am going to be kind to every living thing Again, This is about respect. To respect the parents of yours, elders, friends, as well as animals. Let this loving feeling glow for other people. You won't ever know. A look, thanks, or maybe a simple gesture is able to end up with a ripple effect.

Keen on Learning More About the Advantages of Reiki? Check out These Resources!

Reiki: Everybody is Doing it! by Tracy Morrow - Many important doctors, artists, musicians as well as celebrities have embraced the advantages Reiki

Exactly how Reiki Helped Me Heal & Find The Purpose of mine by Michelle Matthews - An inspiring story of utilizing Reiki to defeat an eating disorder as well as an unhealthy relationship Can Reiki Heal Deep Rooted Suffering and also Pain? by Taryn Walker - An essential read which draws a distinction between curing as well as healing

A Reiki Practitioner is but one who's attuned to the life force energy after which will continue to invite the power in - to not ensure that it stays, but to give out. Think of a Reiki Master as the place or maybe the hollow bone that enables the healing energy to run through them to anywhere healing is desired and or even required.

Be sure you check with an experienced Reiki Master. You will want to work with an experienced whose experience as well as education enables them to perform Reiki properly. It's vital that you really feel a sense and a connection of trust with the Reiki Practitioner of yours, whether you opt to see a proactive Reiki session or maybe a distant Reiki session. Do not hesitate to ask questions! An effective Reiki Practitioner is going to be pleased to reply to or maybe address any concerns or questions you might have as this really helps to produce the feeling of loyalty as well as the comfort which is so necessary to have a good experience. You will want to determine the way the session is going to progress and if you have to do anything to cook.

You will find a few things you are able to do to help make for the Reiki session of yours. The most crucial thing to keep in mind is you would like to feel at ease and relaxed. Wearing loose fitting garments is perfect. Make an effort to refrain from drinking caffeinated drinks and consuming sugary foods the morning of the Reiki session of yours in case in any way possible.

It's a really great practice to drink lots of water the day of the Reiki session of yours. Drinking water is a conductor of electricity and can make it possible to boost the pace of the Reiki energy to run through your actual physical, spiritual and emotional/mental bodies to give off help and blockages to detox as well as balance the chakras of yours.

Both in-person and remote, most Reiki sessions survive between sixty and ninety minutes. Some Reiki masters use a proactive approach with gentle touch, while others hardly ever touch the clients of theirs at all. Understanding what to anticipate will assist you completely relax as well as benefit from the therapy as it occurs.

It is crucial that you realize that the individual getting the Reiki also regulates it. The individual who channels the Reiki doesn't stop the individual who receives the treatment. In reality, the individual receiving treatment remedies him or herself. This is since the individual getting the Reiki takes the quantity of energy needed. This is not accomplished from the conscious mind but a greater level that knows what is best. This part of the brain additionally decides how you can make use of the Reiki energy. As an outcome, the individual channeling Reiki power doesn't handle it and so cannot cause damage. Reiki actually carries a built in protection system against bad energy.

Is Reiki Safe?

Indeed, Reiki is a safe and natural method to heal the body. It is spiritual healing practices that may be used via a professional, but self healing techniques will also be readily available for those who cannot find a specialist in the area of theirs.

Reiki was proven working nicely for the majority of maladies, and may be utilized in conjunction with some other methods, both therapeutic and medical, to market recovery or even alleviate unwanted side effects.

Anyone is able to learn Reiki for self healing purposes, including kids as well as the elderly, as age as well as health state does not affect the capability to practice. Special background or no credentials have to get the needed training. Virtually all it requires is approximately ten hours of personal education from a Reiki practitioner. Usually, these classes are instructed in groups, along with a nominal fee is charged to blanket the class. You do not need any specific knowledge of bioenergy or health care. You'll just have the ability to find out from a professional Reiki master, thus in case you understand a person who practices, question them who taught them. Research into the background of theirs to ensure they're credible adequate to train you.

Religion has spiritual elements, and although Reiki is spiritual, there's no religion. You're not needed in order to have confidence in anything particular to learn Reiki or even to get it to work for you. It is going to work whether you feel it in or perhaps not. The religious part of

Reiki indicates everyone must live as well as act in tactics that promote harmony with each other, an almost culturally common belief.

With Reiki's self healing methods, you are able to apply the methods on your own personal body to alleviate a selection of problems, including: pain relief, anxiety and stress, along with a variety of persistent health issues. Understanding how to work with Reiki on yourself guarantees you are never ever left alone being helpless and out of hand once again.

Chapter 4: Reiki Initiation

Before proceeding any further the reader should know that Reiki is an evolving discipline, having many branches growing from the traditional Reiki developed a century ago.

In consequence there are many schools of Reiki claiming their own point of view on the initiation process. But beside the differences and tones, Reiki remains consistent in terms of core beliefs.

All ways of practicing Reiki target to connect our existence to the higher form of vital energy existing in the Universe.

It is very important to know from the beginning that Reiki is a discipline based on initiation. You can't claim be able to understand and practice Reiki by reading a book or by gathering theoretical knowledge from any other outside source. As the learning curve may become obstructed by the incapacity to evolve spiritually, the person in pursuit of initiation needs the guidance of a Reiki master.

Patience and taking things easy are also essential for embarking in the journey to become a Reiki initiate. Forget about fast results we are used from our speed-paced lifestyle.

Reiki is mostly about slowing down and concentrating on each step along the way.

The ability to access Reiki is conferred following a precise procedure called initiation, something that could be compared to a fine tuning, in which the teacher support its students to access the universal vital force.

Reiki Usui's method has two pillars: the daily practice of self-treatment (applying palms over different parts of your own body, in a certain order) and a daily conduit based on the five principles.

Each Reiki practitioner is initiated by a Reiki master, who was himself initiated and taught directly by another master Reiki, and so on, in an unbroken line, up towards Mikao Usui.

This process of initiation is taught only to those who reach the level of teacher / master. Other practitioners (Level 1 and level 2) are able to access Reiki but are not able to initiate someone else.

Initiation in Reiki cannot be done remotely and direct personal contact between the teacher and student should be made. The initiation procedure involves an information exchange at an energetic level.

It can be also considered to be a journey within and outside the self, a better understanding of its limits and shape. Because every person is unique, every session of initiation and every journey are also unique and personalized. A session is usually restricted to one hour, one hour and a half, depending of the level at which initiation is made.

Usui Reiki, also called traditional Reiki, has four degrees and each requires a separate approach on the initiation process. The fourth level is the level at which you can consider yourself to be a master.

This first level of Reiki has the role of making a short and superficial introduction to the energetic field that will later be explored. The vital energy is perceived at a coarse "resolution" and can be portrayed as a thin, invisible mist of water everywhere around us and inside ourselves. Students learn to communicate with the mineral, plant and animal kingdom using this energetic veil as a common denominator, able to minimize differences we would otherwise consider impossible to surpass.

Reiki is believed to be a universal language, glue for the fabric of the world. The established communication can take many forms, depending on the desired level (energetic, informational, and even spiritual).

After initiation for the first level of Reiki, the practitioner can do only self-treatment. In implementing self-treatment, hand positions are simple and intuitive. In principle, they travel from top to bottom, following the seven chakras, on the front and on rear of the body. Hands can also be applied on painful places.

After being initiated for the first level, the student receives the ability to activate its palms for a higher efficiency. The symbols of Reiki are also revealed to him. Reiki describes the symbols as keys able to unlock, modulate and amplify new levels of energy.

Level 2 of initiation allows the practitioner to remove negative energies from spaces and objects, purify crystals and energize water. At this level the initiated Reiki student is able to make extend its abilities beyond direct contact, making room for remote influencing. This is done mainly trough amplification and allows the creation of protection fields, which act as shields for any negative influences and could serve a house or person.

The second level helps us better know ourselves and better isolate the self. Connecting at this level provide an increase channel for the flowing energy to enter our system. Initiation for the second Reiki level is usually followed by an extended process of purification, for both the soul and the body.

Finishing the second level of Reiki initiation can be considered done when you get close to our true inner self and you become able to live in full consciousness. At this point you have full control over your emotions and you can chose to eliminate tension and worries.

Although Reiki initiation is usually done in the company of a master, from a certain point on, it's all left to you. You will need to win the battle between your old self and the new one emerging.

Reiki traditionally reserves the third level for the degree of master. But no anyone can truly reach the level and commitment and understanding necessary to become a master.

Beside all the courses and guides claiming to take you through all the stages in a record time, Reiki is about finding your true call. Not all Reiki initiates will hear that call well enough to become masters.

This level is usually reserved only for personality enhancement and the initiated entering the third stage of Reiki needs to teach others and confront their problems and blockages. Reiki, like any other holistic practice, is based on cyclicality and reciprocity.

The students are those who help the teacher adapt and perfection its techniques, allowing him to ultimately become a master. His methods should become general solutions for the problems of daily concern.

A Reiki master should never give factual solutions, the same way there is no perfect recipe on how to live. He is only committed to teach Reiki knowledge and live its life in terms with Reiki energy.

For a student wanting to benefit as much as possible from the Reiki learning experience, a few instructions could turn out to be very useful. First of all, try to delimit yourself from any disturbing concern and be fully present at the course. The day should revolve around the few hours dedicated for the Reiki initiation. Allow plenty of time to arrive at your appointment without being in a hurry. It is always better to walk towards the location the Reiki session will take place and visualize that walk as part of your spiritual awakening, something close to a walkabout.

Always dress in the clothes you feel most comfortable in and leave behind any desire to impress. If you are targeting to get closer to your inner self, it is a good idea to allow your true personality at surface. Also, limit or completely eliminate vice and any form of excess towards your body and senses.

Reiki values include simplicity and living life at a slower, more profound pace. Waiting for Reiki lesson with enthusiasm and optimism is the best way to open your mind and heart.

Knowledge is always more easy to assimilate for those who do not fear or reject it. Reiki is not about clinching to performance and being competitive. Reiki is about cooperation and honesty, first towards your master and finally towards yourself.

If you have chosen to follow the initiation process expect to tear down some self-imposed limits and limiting beliefs. Again, this should not be seen in terms of competitiveness and progress, but more in terms of self-development, a growing that takes place inside and it's hard to be visible from the exterior.

Chapter 5: The Religious Myths Continue

So the myths that have been set up by these religious bodies continue on unabated. Sure, they are modifying some of their dogma, but this is because they're having to.

They are losing punters, their life-blood, in droves.

It'd be nice to think that religion is changing, growing and developing out of some kind of spiritual enlightenment, but unfortunately it's purely economic.

It is not, therefore, in their interests for you to leave their religion.

It never has been.

They will threaten you with all kinds of punishments that will be meted out by a harsh and unforgiving God. For All That Is, it seems, will only play ball with you, if you play ball with All That Is.

The Supreme Being will only be loving, caring and understanding if you do precisely as it says. It will not be best pleased if you try to do things your own way and will punish you mightily.

Let's look at that more closely

Now come on.

First of all the religion tells you that you will only be looked after by All That Is if you adhere to the doctrines as put forward by their religion.

The only One True Religion, of course – but they all tell you that don't they?

Then they say that this wonderful, loving, compassionate all powerful, Supreme Being of theirs - The Only One True God of course...

...but they all tell you that as well, don't they? - will punish you for all eternity if you don't comply.

Does this really make any sense?

Does this almighty being not appear to be acting suspiciously like...

'The Devil'?

The absolute antithesis of everything All That Is - is supposed to represent.

Well we don't know about you, but it sure does sound like ol' Nick to us. You see, to us, All That Is represents love, life, freedom and joy.

Pure love - eternal life - absolute freedom -unlimited joy.

Anything else is a lie made up by man.

So let's be clear. The long and the short of it is this...

The present understanding of God's Will and God's Laws etc. comes mostly from one source — Religion. These religions claim to have got their information directly from The Supreme Being, but usually through human intermediaries.

In other words we are supposed to believe in what other people said happened to them, hundreds of years ago.

We are supposed to believe that these few special individuals were the only ones capable of communicating with All That Is. And accept without question that no one else was, is or ever will be capable of doing the same - ever again.

Well, excuse us for saying so. But does that make any sense at all?

Is that really acceptable to you?

Religions are at fault

We're sorry but to us it's quite clear.

It's the religions that are at fault here, not All That Is. The religions do not represent the word of God, they only say that they do, and they have hoodwinked too many people for quite long enough!

You see, religion is one of the foremost institutions for removing, suppressing and controlling every single drop of you and your divine power.

If you are at all religious, please understand that we're not having a go at your particular religion. No, we're having a go at all the organised religions...

...each and every one of them!

There's probably not one single religion on the face of this planet, which seeks to empower you to the point of God head.

They all seek to control you and keep you in fear and bondage.

And, incidentally, most religions spring from the same root too.

In other words almost every religion that people are following today developed from, or has derived elements from, another religion that came before it.

There are no truly unique religions and they're all manmade as we've already said. Yes, we would have to agree that as everyone is a part of All That Is then every religion would have to have been divinely inspired. But they've all been corrupted by mans desire to dominate and control.

Even the ones, which began with noble intentions, have succumbed to the distortions of their later leaders.

And here's another interesting fact - most of them were derived from a worship of the sun, yes, even Christianity.

What is required is clarity.

An understanding of whom and what Infinite Consciousness is, which comes from within each and every individual.

Look, you have not, do not and never will have the need for an intermediary to communicate with All That Is, because

All That Is - is inside you right now.

Because,

All That Is - is you - and you are All That Is.

All That Is does not create all the atrocities occurring in our world today, we do. We've chosen to experience these things and All That Is/We, have given ourselves the freedom to have these experiences.

It cannot happen any other way. All That Is will never over-rule us, because it cannot. Our will is its will.

Now let this really sink in...

Our will *is God*'s will

because

God's will is *our* will.

Back to the beginning again

Now let's just go back again to the beginning of time. To that place we are becoming more familiar with.

If you've really tried the exercise we asked you to try, you will know that it's not possible to imagine that there has ever been a time when you were not.

There's never been a time of complete nothingness.

Okay, so stretch with this a little, and bring your umbrellas if you need to.

If you can accept that there must have been a beginning.

A somewhere, a sometime, when it all began!

You can do this can't you? Yes? Good.

What, or who, do you think was there at that moment?

Yes, we know this can conjure up images of chickens and eggs, but lay that aside for a minute. (Apologies for the awful pun).

Is it easier to imagine that there was some kind of other energy there, along with you, rather than some kind of inanimate object?

Is it easier to imagine that this energy had some kind of intelligence or consciousness rather than being inert?

Yes, we know this isn't easy, but what we're trying to do is get you to a place where you can allow the possibility.

For most people who've given this subject some serious consideration...

...and many people have, their conclusions - albeit probably not conclusive - are usually along the lines of, it must have started somewhere.

But if you really can't accept that there was a beginning, and that there must have been some sort of energy there.

What else is there, you can accept?

Most scientists put forward the theory of the Big Bang as being the beginning of the universe.

In fact this theory is becoming the generally accepted reality.

Others don't agree at all. But the thing is, they all agree on one thing – there must have been a beginning.

And, as we've said, it's very chicken and egg, but we think it all boils down (not a pun) to just the one question...

Did the beginning have structure and intelligence behind it, or was it just a totally random, chance event?

Our belief system

Now, we've gone back to this point, and meditated on it many, many times. And our understanding, drawn from these experiences, is that it all started with the energy of consciousness.

This consciousness had great intelligence, wisdom and compassion.

It was all that there was, and it knew that it was all that there was.

And because we are unable to imagine a time when we were not, and are also unable to imagine a time when we will not ever be, we know that we were, and are, part of this consciousness.

For you, this knowing may not yet be.

But we hope to change that.

You see, our own journey to this realisation also originally started out in hope.

We hoped that what we were feeling and understanding was true.

And, after a while, this hope changed into a tentative belief that it was true.

This belief eventually, after much trial and error, became a knowing.

And, we now hope to engender within you this same kind of knowing.

Back to the beginning, once more

So, back to this conscious energy source at the beginning of time once again. (We hope you will forgive us for all these happy returns but it was, after all, your birthday).

As we've said, you existed as a part of this energy and everything was incredibly marvellous.

You were all there was and you were magnificent.

Now being all there was and being incredibly marvellous was all very well and good, but it was also just a bit too conceptual...

A tad too much on the theoretical side for your liking!

In fact, it was bordering on the all talk no action way of life – a little like trying to learn to ride a bike just by reading a book about it.

Which is not very practical because it leaves you thinking you know how to do it until you get on the bike, then whoops, you're instantly upside down, in a heap.

You wanted to experience what it was like to be magnificent. You wanted to ride that bike, you wanted to feel that wind, feel what it was like to be upside down.

You wanted to get down and boogie a little.

So how do you do it? How do you get out there and start experiencing things?

Now remember, you are all there is and, 'out there' doesn't exist, yet. There's nothing at all that exists which is not a part of you.

You are the everything of everything, the whole kit and caboodle.

It might also be worth mentioning at this point, that you're also the everything of that which is not, as well.

Chapter 6: The Reiki Ideals

Years after founding and developing the natural healing system of Reiki, Dr Usui decided, during a meditation, to regulate five principles to the Reiki System in order to bring in spiritual balance and to help people to consciously settle on to improve their way of life and themselves. The objective of including the Five Reiki Principles was to instigate students of Reiki with a responsibility to take an active part in their own healing process. Dr Usui also considered that practicing the Reiki Ideals would facilitate with certainty the progress of Reiki Healing and thus encourage and promote lasting results. According to Dr Usui, the active commitment that the individual takes to improve themselves in life further assists in completing the natural healing system. The Usui Reiki Ideals also act as guidelines on how a person can live a congenial life and practice worthy virtues for their own inherent value.

The Five Reiki Principles

At a certain period in his life, Dr Usui worked in Kyoto, at the beggar's colony, healing and attuning patients (mostly beggars) to the Reiki System. It goes without saying that he did that free of charge. By doing so, Dr Usui expected that Reiki would soon work as a medium towards getting the poor and the beggarly people out of their miserable conditions and encourage them to turn over a new leaf and start life afresh. Dr Usui counted on the fact that Reiki would aid the deprived people in a time of need and guide them towards having a clearer understanding of themselves and of their surroundings. Du Usui put his trust in the conviction that Reiki would ultimately help them emerge from their lowly conditions and seek work in order to earn an honest living. With this vision and prospect Dr Usui initiated and taught many destitute, beggars and homeless people.

However, after a few years, when Dr Usui came back to Kyoto to find out how his Reiki channels were faring, he was bitterly disappointed to see that nothing had really changed in the area. He was displeased to find out that almost all of his Reiki channels were still begging to earn a living. Dr Usui then realized that something might have gone wrong in the way of his "giving" Reiki to them. He went and questioned some of them about why they were still begging and why they were still poor. The Reiki channels told him that while they got healed from their diseases through Dr Usui's Reiki System of healing, they were nevertheless unable to alter their way of living. They even went to the extent of telling Dr Usui that they would have preferred being sick and in their former condition than healed and healthy because people now refused to give them money because they looked in good physical shape. To his utter disappointment, Dr Usui realized there and then that while his system of healing had nursed back to health his patients' bodies, their minds and spirit still remained diseased and afflicted.

That was when Dr Usui decided to add the Five Reiki Principles to his System of healing. He was assertive that without those Five Reiki Principles his Reiki Healing System would remain incomplete.

Dr Usui also came to the conclusion that anything given freely could never be of much value to the one who received it. On the other hand, something received against something else was sure to be used intelligently and cleverly. In other words, when someone badly needed something and went to the extent of buying it for themselves, they were sure of taking great care of it and use it carefully. So, Dr Usui came to a conclusion there and then that there should be an 'exchange' of Energy between the Giver and the Receiver of Reiki.

'Just for Today...'

However, the five Reiki Principles of Dr Usui are not generally easy to follow. It is not possible for a normal human being to suddenly get rid of all his worries overnight or to suddenly have a control over his anger. This is the reason why Dr

Usui started each sentence of his Five Reiki Principles with the phrase: '*Just for today*'.

Dr Usui's Five Reiki Principles are as follows:

Just for today, I will not be angry.

Just for today I will not worry.

Just for today I will do my work honestly.

Just for today I will be grateful.

Just for today I will be kind to all living beings.

The idea behind the phrase '*just for today*' is that, normally, it is impossible for a person to shed all their negative feelings all of a sudden and for good. However, it may be easier to start with a little at a time. Therefore, trying to get rid of one negative feeling for just a day seems an easier exercise and may as well work for the one trying it. While Dr Usui commends us to pursue the Five Reiki Principles throughout our life, he also shows us the way to go about it which is by dozing it little by little in our existence until we become attuned to them and thus cure our mind and body.

I believe that each day in the life of a living being is in itself an important portion of a lifetime. Can we not live just a single day meeting the requirements of just one of these Five Reiki Principles? And then it becomes so much easier if we chose ourselves our Principle for the Day. For example, let us decide as we wake up in the morning that, just for today we are going to control our anger. From there we move up, adjusting our position for the whole day and remaining totally honest to our resolution, to ourselves and to those around us. If we are successful, then that's it, we are done! We feel great that we have finally lived through a whole, *'anger-less'* day which is in itself wonderful, both for us and for those around us!

Therefore, choose your Reiki Principle for the Day and live it fully, honestly, day in and day out without faltering. If you falter (it's human), then try again, improving and ameliorating as you go. Remember, whether you are a Giver or a Receiver of Reiki, the Five Reiki Principles are mandatory if you desire Reiki to heal you at all levels in life.

The Essence of the Reiki Ideals

The nucleus of the Five Reiki Principles helps a person understand and assimilate the heart of the matter—the very essence inherent in the short phrases.

To Live for Today

It is important for an individual to practice daily all the Five Reiki Ideals. With each moment of Reiki practice, you will learn to live each moment and, as a result, each day over every inch and thoroughly. 'Living for the Day' is a continuous process that will determine and complete your Reiki learning and healing in the long run.

To Let Go of Anger

Anger, if it feels completely normal as it is a human emotion, more than often gets out of control, becoming destructive in the overall quality of your life. When you are angry, your life energy becomes disturbed. Anger hurts not only others to whom they are targeted, but also your own self eventually. Learn to live without intense emotional responses bringing in a lot of peace and quiet around you. With Reiki, you will learn to recover the balance of your emotions and your mind. Therefore, according to the Reiki Ideals, you must control your anger before it controls you.

To Trust

Unnecessary fears and worries can be of no good, for they can only embrangle your life energy. The Usui Reiki Ideals will help you trust the Universe of which you are a part. By trusting, by having complete confidence in the Universe and by never doubting for a minute, you will learn to be at your very best at whatever you do. Let the Universe take care of the rest. This will allow you to live each day with peace of mind, equanimity and quiescence. Once you begin to trust the Universe, to all that exists around you, your attunement to the Reiki Energy will become whole and strong.

To Be Grateful

Show your appreciation and be filled with gratitude when you receive the benefits of the Reiki Healing System. By being thus thankful, you and your family will naturally become the right recipients of the Reiki Energy experienced. Through your attunement with the Great Energy of the Universe, you will also learn to be grateful for every other thing you acquire in your life. Never take anything for granted and work constantly to better yourself.

To Be Active

The saying goes: *'Idle hands do the devils work'*. A lazy mind is disadvantageous for any person. It is only through continued learning and practice of the Five Reiki Ideals that one is able to grow as an individual. As you progress in life,

bettering yourself each day, your bond with the Life-energy also develops and expands. Therefore, be filled with activity and be always on the move. You can only benefit by being physically and mentally active. It is the spiritual medicine for all illness.

To be kind

To be kind is what we should aspire to be in life. Being kind is the cornerstone of life—the most important thing we are taught by our elders since our childhood.

Being kind to everything around us in the Universe is even more important than being ambitious or successful.

Once you step in the world of Reiki, you cannot help but develop a sense of oneness with the Universe and everything which forms part if it. It is said: *"Be kind to strangers for they may be Angels in disguise."* You will learn that the Reiki System of Healing also means practice of good heartedness, love and compassion. There is no real distinction between you and others. Every living entity is endowed with life, with soul. Everyone is the same in the sense that they are all unique. We are all unique. So, in general, we are all the same even if our individual qualities are different. However, being kind also means that one should be genuinely kind not only to others but also to oneself. Reiki teaches us that we are all equal on the spiritual level because we are all connected although we are each uniquely different on a physical and mental level.

Reiki is Not a Business!

When people consult Reiki practitioners, they go to them, often as a last resort, to find solutions to their difficult situations, to obtain results and help for their illnesses and their predicaments and to find a way to their roadblocks. The sole aim of the true Reiki Practitioner is to give full attention to the seeker and help them improve over time, lighten their load and lend their Reiki hand to lead them to self-confidence, renewed health and self-trust. The Reiki Healer feels that it is the phenomenon of Divine love which passes through them into another. Reiki is miraculous because miracles do happen during the Reiki healing process.

However, over the years we have also witnessed cases where some unscrupulous Reiki practitioners go to the extent of breaking the promise of a developing Reiki practice and turn it into a dishonest and conscienceless business.

Reiki is not a business! It is a vocation but not commerce. The give and take in Reiki should be truthful, upright and honest exchange between Giver and Receiver. It should not be negotiation, bargaining and merchandising.

And yet, we have been taking cognizance of emerging unprincipled Reiki practitioners who are making use of Dr Usui's noble and unselfish experience to make money hand over fist and fill their insatiable treasure chests.

Dr Usui applied himself selflessly in the Kyoto slums and he did it on a purely experimental basis in those days which never involved money. But there a few out there who, in the name of Dr Usui's Reiki healing System, want to justify their sky high fees for their Reiki training and healing. Consequently we are also taking cognizance of the fact that Reiki is more and more becoming accessible only to the rich. Those disadvantaged and deprived, who perhaps deserve Reiki the most, are very often having difficulties accessing this God-sent healing blessing.

I certainly don't mean here that Reiki therapists, in the course of their practice, should deny themselves to needs to make a living out of their Reiki practice. I don't deny the fact that a Reiki practitioner, just like any other therapist, needs to earn an honest living. But I feel some Reiki practitioners, in their own best interest and for their own good reputation, should know where to draw the line between Reiki practice and Reiki business. Reiki is invaluable. Charging patients and students exaggerated sums of money in exchange of healing and training goes against the very principles of Reiki and devaluates the spiritual nature of this noble Healing System. In other words it defeats the very purpose of Reiki.

As it is, Reiki therapists know quite well that Dr Usui never used the word 'money' while describing the 'exchange' of Energy between the Giver and the Receiver of Reiki. According to Dr Usui, Reiki healing was very much like the barter system—that ancient method of exchange long before money was invented. In those days people exchanged services and goods in return of other services. In the same way according to Dr Usui, for a Reiki healing, any other thing than money could be most welcome as an exchange. For example, a candle, some flowers, some incense sticks from the patient could be most welcome. And in cases where the patient had really nothing else to offer, then a prayer, a 'thank you' or even, simply, a grateful smile would be most welcome.

Attunement to Reiki

In order to make use of Reiki one needs to be attuned to the Universal Energy or to the Life-force Energy. Attunement to Reiki should *always* be conducted by a skilled and trained Reiki Teacher/Master. Reiki cannot be learned on your own or even from a book. The traditional spiritual ceremony helps you connect with the Energy-Source of Reiki. I would even compare this Reiki attunement ceremony to a 'rebirth' for the one being initiated to Reiki. Many things can happen during and after an attunement. Once you are attuned to the Reiki Energy-Source, you will become aware of your self-empowerment. You will be able to use energy in your own life and on those around you for a continuous healing process of the body, mind, and spirit.

Chapter 7: The Principles And Pillars Of Reiki

Within most practices of a healing nature, there are usually some specific guidelines and rules of understanding. In order to form a structure to understand and identify the reality of your practice, you must first build the foundation of that structure. To put it plainly, there are principles and pillars to the practice of Reiki that will give you the overall structure of how to perform Reiki healing treatments and remind you of why you are doing it in the first place.

The reality of Reiki is that it is a focus that unifies us with our inherent quality as humans to be a source of love and light, and to unite us with all forms of energy available in the Universe we. In order to understand your true nature, there are concepts that can be meditated on to help you realize the nature of your internal integrity and power.

The Principles and Pillars of Reiki are what Mikao Usui developed as a response to his Buddhist teachings and his own personal awakening through the origination of Reiki practices. When you see these principles and pillars, imagine that they are like a mission statement and the basis of how to heal from the inside out.

The Principles of Reiki

The Principles of Reiki are an incredibly simple set of words to help you understand that there is no need to over-complicate the logic of the Universe and the energy of life as we know it on Earth. The structure of the Principles is outlined to make it easy for you to repeat them to yourself like a mantra.

Many Reiki Masters and practitioners will use these principles in their meditations and prior to performing Reiki on a client or even on themselves. These attitudes and beliefs help you do away with any harmful or negative thoughts so that you can keep your channels clear to be a healing conduit of light energy and Universal love. You don't have to memorize them right away;

you can write them down and keep them in your pocket, or keep them somewhere you will see them every day until they are familiar to you.

Reflect upon these principles so that they add more meaning to your life and your healing journey. The Reiki Principles are:

Just for today, I will not worry.

Just for today, I will not be angry.

Just for today, I will do my work honestly.

Just for today, I will give thanks for my many blessings.

Just for today, I will be kind to every living thing.

The five Reiki Principles are a standard reality for anyone who wants to act as a channel of healing energy. If you are intending to help not only yourself but other people as well, you have to adhere to a certain level of principle in order to be effective while using Reiki as a healing tool and treatment method. Let's look at the principles one by one so that you understand what each of them means.

Just for today, I will not worry.

This principle says that if you are in a state of worry you cannot heal easily and with openness in your heart. If you are in a state of worry, you are looking at things with narrow eye-sight and are not able to see a bigger picture. Reiki is a bigger picture and asks you to leave your doubts and worries behind, even if only for today so that you can learn to move beyond them and see the light of love that flows through your hands in into your very own heart.

Just for today, I will not be angry.

This principle says that anger is a source of negativity that will cause you a deeper and more painful wound. If you are carrying energy in your heart you will not be able to effectively channel Reiki energy for healing. It is not a matter of just saying that you are not angry anymore; it is understanding why you have anger if you do and discovering how to release it and heal the source of it. The words "just for today" ask you to try every day to heal the source of any anger you may feel, no matter the cause and that it is more important to live a life without anger than to live with it in your heart and cause further pain to yourself and others.

Just for today, I will do my work honestly.

This principle says that Reiki is an act of truth and that you must have honesty in order to act as a channel of light and love. If you are utilizing the healing power of Reiki to manipulate others or work on yourself in ways that can affect you negatively, then you are not being honest with your truth. There are people all over the world who are living dishonestly with themselves, afraid to be clear and direct with what is right and what is wrong. You cannot use Reiki to manipulate others or it will cause you deeper pain and harder struggles. You must work with yourself and other people as honestly as is possible.

Just for today, I will give thanks for my many blessings.

This principle says that the most effective way to remain a positive channel of light, love, and healing Reiki life-force is to offer your gratitude to the Universal truth of all things. Gratitude is a powerful force and many of us forget to offer our thanks for everything that we have, right now, at this moment. So often we are striving for what is far out ahead of us and forget to notice what is right in front of us. The power of thankfulness and gratitude is a reflection of Universal Love consciousness and is a part of the awakening and the enlightenment journey. You can heal your own wounds through simple acts of daily gratitude and bridge the gap between what you think you are supposed to be with what you already are.

Just for today, I will be kind to every living thing.

This principle says that you are in an awareness that we are always in responsibility to the whole Universe, not just to ourselves, or even just other human beings. Every dog, every spider, every lamppost, tree, every rock, every forest, every waterfall, and sea must be loved by us all. Reiki is a powerful force of love and light and asks for us to be clear about our intentions when we are working with this powerful force. You can be loving and kind to all matter, even the fork you use to eat your supper or the slug in your garden who won't leave your flowers alone. The aspect of kindness is imperative to be a channel of Reiki and so must be considered every day that you are practicing.

The five principles are the foundation of your understanding of Reiki and what it asks of you if you are going to be an open channel of healing light and love for yourself and others. These principles are a very simple structure to be built upon and as you proceed into the next section, you will discover what the Pillars of Reiki will do to support your practice.

The Pillars of Reiki

The Pillars are the next layer of the structure of Reiki, giving additional form to helping you live through the practice. They are based on specific concepts of Buddhism, learned by Usui at the time of his enlightenment and years of study. They contribute to the Reiki Principles by giving meaning to them through the body, mind, and spirit. They are meditations and hand positions to help you achieve focus, balance, and inner wisdom from the heart.

Pillar 1: Gassho

Gassho means "two hands coming together." In Buddhist practices, a Gassho is performed regularly to signify a specific meaning. The simplicity of a single hand gesture speaks volumes and illuminates the ascended self and how you are experiencing yourself and your true oneness. The Gassho is the palms pressed together, as if in prayer and held in a variety of ways or used in specific meditation to attain a certain spiritual goal.

A gassho is a symbol of respect and states that you are one with everyone and everything no matter their race, religion, cultural background, orientation, or affiliation. It is a posture of Universal truth, love, and oneness. There are a variety of gasshos that are performed and you will learn many in your explorations depending on greatly you choose to explore the realities of Buddhism. For the practices of Reiki, you only need to know two: the formal gassho and Mu-Shin gassho.

The formal gassho can be performed in practices you are performing on yourself or others before treatment. It is considered useful for rituals, religious services, and ceremonies, but can be used any time you need it. Here are the steps for the formal gassho:

Place the palms together at heart level.

The arms should be extended out and away from the body so that the elbows are slightly bent.

Point your fingers at a 45-degree angle.

Keep them at the level of the heart, extending light and Universal life-force through you and out from you.

This gassho signifies devotion to spirit and the divine. It expresses reverence and respect for creation and the energy of the Universe while expressing the same reverence for those around us.

The Mu-Shin gassho is slightly different. Mu-shin means "no mind" and is a common attitude for meditation and prayer that states, "we are one and I respect you and all things." Here are the steps for the Mu-Shin gassho:

Put both of your hands, palm, to palm, at heart level.

Pull your hands close the chest and connect them to your heart center so that they are touching you (instead of extended out like in the formal gassho).

Arrange your hands so that your fingers are pointing up toward your chin.

Meditate, breathe, prepare.

This gassho can be used in the midst of your self-healing treatments, or other meditations, as well as during any healing experiences you are sharing with other people. This simple pillar has a powerful way of connecting you and grounding you into your power and healing abundance. You can use either gassho to support your healing work and your life-force energy.

Pillar 2: Reiji-Ho

Reiji-Ho is a prayer or a meditation that is often used for distance healing work. When you are asking to connect with someone who is far away from you, or even to your past or future self, you can use this Reiki Pillar to relax your mind and set your intentions. It helps you to be more directly and clearly guided in your use of Reiki. Rather than trying to guess where to go with your healing hands and energy, you are **shown** when you open yourself with this meditation.

Use Mu-Shin gassho and meditate on your energy by asking for Reiki to flow through you. Ask for it three times. Wait for the rise of the energy and then move forward.

Bring your gassho up to your third eye (above and between the eyebrows) and ask for your health and recovery on every level if it is needed. You may also be asking for someone else, in which case you would state their name in your mind. This act will ask the Reiki energy to flow where it is most needed. Ask the energy to guide your hands to the places that need the most healing energy.

Allow your hands to be pulled and pushed wherever they may be guided to go. It may take time and practice and you will find the pull very clearly when you release yourself and allow the energy to flow through you freely. You may be in this third phase for a while as you are working with your own practices, or on someone else, but usually not longer than 1 hour.

Complete the Reiji-Ho pillar with Mu-Shin for as long as you need for disconnection from the experience.

Again, this pillar is helpful for the self as well as others and can be performed before any healing treatment. It will help you respond more clearly and directly by being guided by the Reiki energy moving forward and through to show you where you need the most healing energy work.

Pillar 3: Chiryo

The third and final Reiki Pillar is another guided meditation to help you find the greatest source of healing need in the self or another.

You will begin at the crown of the head, holding the dominant hand above it until you feel the inspiration from Reiki energy to move in a direction. You will be shown where to go to relieve any issues.

Usually, your hands will hover over, or be placed in the area they were drawn to until the source of the issue is relieved and your hands are ready to move to the next placement.

You will be shown by Reiki where to move next. It feels very intuitive and you have to be fully open and receptive as a conduit of healing life-force energy in order for this pillar to work for you.

It can take a lot of practice, or if you are already attuned to a second level, then it may feel a lot easier because your channels are already more open, clear, and attentive.

You may also use a series of breaths that will usually be taught by your Reiki Master in practicing and learning this pillar of Reiki. Breath is a valuable tool for remaining open to the flow of Reiki through you. Your breath clears the body, mind, and spirit and will further aid and assist your openness while performing this meditation.

All of the pillars are simple and easy to practice. Together with the principles, you have the structure of Reiki and how it is asking you to be available to the service of healing yourself and others. Learn these techniques and tools and it will set you up for exactly what you need in your Reiki healing experience.

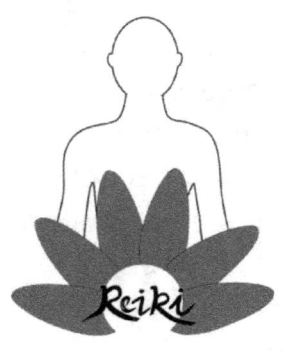

Chapter 8: Practicing Reiki

Every person who engages in Reiki practice will experience it differently. This is because your experience depends on a number of factors, including your commitment to Reiki, your faith in the spiritual energy, and how you set the intent before the session. While everyone experiences it differently, the practice will be almost identical. This chapter will teach you everything that you need to know to perform a successful Reiki session.

Reiki and the Chakras

If you have ever done healing yoga or meditation, you may already know a little bit about chakras. If not, the basic definition of a chakra is an energy center. These centers exist at 7 key points of the human body. They are used to help transmit the flow of energy. When you practice Reiki, focusing on the chakras will allow the Reiki energy to fill your body easily and effectively.

Imagine the chakras of the body as a vertical tube of energy that flows straight up and down the body. Each of the seven chakras is located along this vertical tube. Read on to learn more.

About Each of the Chakras

The **Root Chakra** (also called the base) is located at the base of your spine. It is the chakra on your body located closest to the earth and it is considered to be linked with grounding to the earth and physical survival. When this chakra is blocked, it can cause defensiveness, fear, paranoia, and procrastination.

The **Navel Chakra** (also called the Sacral Chakra) can be found between your navel and the base of your spine. It is related very closely to emotion and represents feelings like sexuality, pleasure, and desire. It is also known to be linked to creativity and procreation. When this chakra is blocked, you may feel sexual guilt, emotional problems, and compulsive behaviors.

The **Solar Plexus Chakra**, like the Navel Chakra, is associated with emotional health. This chakra is located above your navel and beneath your rib cage, in the solar plexus area. It is known to be the root of feelings like anger, personal power, joy, and laughter, and also your levels of ambition and sensitivity. When this chakra is blocked, it may cause frustration, anger, and a lack of direction.

The **Heart Chakra** is considered the house of the soul, as it is the center of peace, harmony, love, and compassion. It is located at the center of your chest, just over from the heart. When this chakra is blocked, you may find immune system troubles, heart and lung illnesses, or even inhumane behaviors.

The **Throat Chakra** is found within the throat. It is known for its strong connection to communication and also as the power house for self-expression and creativity. It encourages healing, purification, and transformation. When this chakra is blocked, it can manifest as creative blocks, communication problems, or dishonesty.

The **Third Eye Chakra** (also called the Brow Chakra) is found just above eye level, at the center of your forehead. It is connected strongly to your spiritual nature and is known as the chakra of perception, knowledge, and questioning. It is also related to internal wisdom and intuition. When this chakra is blocked, you may face depression, a lack of foresight, and selective memory problems.

The **Crown Chakra** is found just above the top of your head. It is connected to both the central nervous system and the cerebral cortex and is considered to be connected to understanding, information, and acceptance. When this chakra is blocked, you may face psychological problems.

Practicing Reiki: Choosing the Chakras to Use

You have two options for Reiki practice, either doing an overall treatment for all of the systems of your body or singling out one or more chakras for individual treatment. Some people also prefer to do an overall treatment once a day and a single chakra at other times, as it is needed throughout the day. This section will teach you what you need to know about both types of practice.

Reiki Practice: Using All of the Chakras

This particular type of Reiki session will take between 15 and 30 minutes, depending on the amount of time that you spend on each area of your body. While using the chakras is especially important for isolating areas, you will use them as a guide, rather than positioning for a total practice. Before you do these, get into position by lying down, however you are most comfortable. You may find that laying on your side or back works very well. Here are the hand positions you will use:

Position 1- Overlap the hands over top the crown of your head.

Position 2- Place one hand on your forehead. Take your second hand and place it between the base of your skull and the crown of your head, on the backside of your head.

Position 3- Rest your hands over both ears.

Position 4- Rest your hands over both eyes.

Position 5- Place one hand on the solar plexus where the rib cage comes to meet and the other on the upper part of your chest.

Position 6- Place your hands on either side of your hips.

Each of these positions should be performed with the palms inward, so that they are touching your body and channeling Reiki energy. Alternatively, you can do a complete Reiki by focusing on each of the individual chakras. For this, you would place the hands on the crown of your head, across your brow, over your throat, in the center of your chest, at the solar plexus, over your navel, and over top of your pelvis.

Hold each position for two to five minutes, depending on how long you would like each session to last. You can decide this beforehand and set a timer to go off. If you do use a timer, however, be sure to choose one that emits a relaxing tone, rather than a harsh ding. You may even be able to find an app for your phone that will allow you to set intervals for the alarm and emits sweet tones.

How to Use a Byosen Scan to Activate the Most Effective Chakras

To do a Boysen scan, you are going to keep your hand palm-side down about 2-3 inches from your body. Lie down and hover your hand down the imaginary vertical line where your chakras are located through your body. Start at the crown and slowly work downward, pausing for a few seconds over each area to notice any changes in the tingling of the Reiki energy or changes in temperature. It is possible you may also feel pain in your palm over the area that needs attention. If you notice any of these changes in an area, see which chakra corresponds. This is the chakra that you should focus on during the session. You can focus on specific areas by only doing Reiki with them or by completing a full session but giving these areas extra attention.

Your goal over the next few weeks should be to practice Reiki every day. This will help you reach toward your long-term goals and give you confidence in your natural abilities. Once you have done this for quite some time, you can further the harmony and peace in your life by working with others. In the next chapter, you will learn how to do just that.

Chapter 9: The Reiki Healing Tool

Physical Reiki enhances the body's inbuilt ability to heal itself. It relieves the body of toxins and poisons and it balances and harmonizes the body to promote wholeness and an overall feeling of wellness. It also helps the body to be aware of its own basic and most pertinent need like the right nutrition, exercise and sleep patterns.

Emotional Reiki directly affects one's emotional energy. It implores them to examine their emotional responses to people and situations and encourages positive emotions like love, care, laughter, happiness, trust, goodwill. It is also known to convert emotional energy into creativity.

Mental Reiki affects one's thinking processes, encouraging them to let go of negative thoughts. It also encourages positivity and serenity. Consequently, this leads to a state of deep relaxation. Reiki works with the energy field to enhance intuitive abilities. It boosts a person's consciousness and self-awareness to help them pursue their personal goals and dreams.

Spiritual Reiki affects the soul and the spirit. It flows into the entire energy body and helps one to love and accept themselves. It also fosters a more tolerant view of mankind, pushing one to accept people as they are, with their different spiritual paths. It fosters love, compassion, tolerance, acceptance and puts one on the path to connecting with the Divine.

Whichever way we look at it, what is very glaring here is taking responsibility for your own health and well-being. Be an active participant in your self-healing. Reiki is not a cure-all technique even though it is very valuable in helping you achieve optimum health. It helps to alienate pain and discomfort but it requires a willingness to allow attitudinal and lifestyle changes so that the healing is whole and permanent.

To practice Reiki, you must take a level of responsibility for your own health. You must be willing and able to respond to the effects of your body's energy being stimulated. You must be willing to come to a better understanding of what your body needs and be able to treat your body with dignity, love, and respect.

Therefore, if you use Reiki every day but continue with habits and lifestyles that are not wholesome for your spiritual, emotional, mental and physical wellbeing, your body will keep on reacting adversely. In other words, Reiki is not invincible. It cannot work until you consciously allow it to.

This is what Reiki First Degree emphasizes — the ability to use Reiki on yourself for self-healing. Reiki moves away blockages within your energy system, slowly making its way through layers of stagnant energy most likely caused by negative thoughts or unhealthy lifestyles which will often come to your mind as memories when you begin Reiki. This "letting go" process is very necessary.

As the memories come, you are given an opportunity to heal and to learn from them. It takes weeks, months and sometimes even years but you will find that you're more vitalized, energetic and happy as it progresses.

Experiencing Reiki Healing

Typically, a client lies fully clothed on a massage table and the Reiki practitioner places his/her hands on or near the client's body. It is important to note here that, Reiki acts under a Divine power and as it works holistically, the energy may not go to work exactly where the practitioner is placing his/her hand. The energy will work on the underlying causes of discomfort in the body, even those that the client is not aware of. An example is, if one is having a stress-induced headache, the ki or life force energy will not just treat the discomfort of a headache but will also go ahead to work on the client's mental state that is causing the headache.

So the Reiki master places his/her hand in a series of hand positions for 2-10 minutes depending on the duration of time for the particular hand position. The entire treatment or session will likely last between 45 minutes to an hour. Depending on the client's condition, he/she may either need to continue the sessions bi-weekly or if they find that they are completely healed in that one session, not at all.

Different people have different Reiki experiences. A lot of people feel a sense of deep relaxation. Others feel a glowing radiance or energy. Others see visions or have an out-of-body experience. At times, when the Reiki Practitioner feels blockages in the chakras, the client may feel an initial heaviness followed by a release and subsequently, a flow of energy.

Chapter 10: Other Reiki Uses

Besides healing and the relief of mental stress, Reiki can also be used in a variety of other ways. In this chapter, we will tackle some of the other common uses for this practice and how you can apply it more to your daily living.

Reiki for Pregnant Women:

Is it safe? This is the first question that any pregnant woman would ask before trying out any kind of therapy during their term. For Reiki, the answer is yes. Both mom and her baby can benefit from the practice's gentle yet effective balancing energies.

The most beneficial thing is that this process is done in an all-natural manner, so there are no risks associated with it at all. Even if you're undergoing other treatments, it will not interfere. Instead, it would help replenish depleted energies and provide comfort through a calming and healing energy. It is not unknown that many pregnant women tend to go through bouts of anxiety during their term. This practice would help with that and soothe the restless spirit.

It is also for them to receive Reiki attunement. In fact, some choose to have their babies attuned to Reiki whilst they are still in the womb. It is a gift whenever it is received or given. And among its teachings is that Reiki is everyone's birthright, therefore, the act of giving is merely a way of awakening it. In other words, it helps us become more in tune to this life force energy that's inside all of us.

Reiki for Babies and Toddlers:

What about for kids? Will Reiki be just as effective and beneficial? Yes, babies and small children too can benefit from it. It is simply instinctual or natural for toddlers as well as babies to be more receptive when it comes to these energies. Parents who have had their offspring attuned to Reiki can attest to the fact that energy almost spontaneously flows to them whenever they are being given the treatment.

As they grow into toddlers or preschoolers, they will need and actually want to be given Reiki. After all, quite like the adults that give it to them, they suffer from mild bouts of stress, and the energies provided by the practice certainly help in calming down that listlessness.

How to give them Reiki?

Of course, conducting a Reiki session with a child isn't the same as treating someone your age or older. The major difference lies in the amount of time allotted for the session itself. A full session for a child would be quite brief when compared to that of an adult's while being no less effective. This is because kids are like Reiki sponges and as mentioned earlier, far more receptive to it than an adult. They don't have the same emotional defenses that many adults do along with the imbalances and blockages which may hinder proper energy flow. And this is also all fortunately good since children tend to want to do a variety of things in so short a time since their attention on things changes easily and often.

When giving your child Reiki, always remember to take cues from them when it comes to ending the session. They may vocalize it or you might notice a restlessness or anxiousness which can happen once they have absorbed enough energy. For kids, 10 to 15 minutes is usually all it takes - compare that to the 60 minutes that an average adult requires, and you'll be able to see the vast difference between energy absorption for both ages.

Reiki for Family Pets:

Reiki can be used during the following:

☐ When they become sick. Reiki would help in facilitating healing and would also comfort them if the symptoms become painful or stressful.

☐ When they undergo any form of trauma. The loving energy that you provide through Reiki can help them get over an event that might have them feeling listless. From moving to a new home, and losing an owner or a sibling - even pets can undergo depression - Reiki could help them cope.

Now, animals would respond differently to Reiki depending on their personality as well as their current condition. If you intend on doing this yourself and not going to a professional, here are a few tips on how you can get started:

☐ Distant Reiki might be better if your pet reacts aggressively towards getting touched. It might be that they're in pain or simply can't stay still for a lengthened period of time.

☐ If your pet allows you to perform hands-on Reiki then make sure you touch them lightly and stop when they begin showing signs of restlessness. Much like young children, the time it takes for them to absorb the energy is far shorter than that of an adult human's.

☐ There are instances wherein your pet would actually approach you, letting you know that they're ready to receive Reiki. This could happen while you're giving the treatment to yourself or to another person. The healing energy attracts them.

☐ Larger animals such as big dogs and horses might require one or more people to simultaneously send love and healing. Teaching your kids and allowing them to participate would be great for this purpose.

The thing about Reiki is that it benefits all living things that move with the life source energy. And contrary to what most people tend to believe, our beloved pets can experience stress too. Be it mentally or physically due to a condition, healing energy would certainly do pets well when stressed.

Reiki for Food:

Just like when praying to give thanks for food, you can also Reiki your meal to get the most from all the nutrients in it. This can also shield you from any impurities or substances that you do not like (e.g., preservatives, fertilizers, artificial additives, hormones, etc.) whether the food is claimed to be organic or not.

To do this, just hold your hands, palm-side down over the food like praying over it. This need not take a long time to do. Just stretch your hands with enough time to visualize and feel all the positive powerful energy flowing into the food.

Reiki for Vitamins, Supplements, and Medications

Similar to meals, you can also apply Reiki to all your vitamins, supplements, and medications if there is a need to take them. In this way you can get the most from all the helpful ingredients, and protect yourself from any substances with potentially harmful side effects especially if taken excessively or when you're not aware if such exist.

To do this, ground and center yourself by breathing deeply, visualizing, and feeling the positive healing energy combining it only with the healing benefits of the medicine while blocking all the side effects. As you do this, hold the whole bottle in both of your hands and begin channeling Reiki. Before ending, picture yourself feeling healthy and happy.

Chapter 11: How To Start Helping Others

Before we go any further, I want everyone to understand that Reiki is not a religion, it was never a religion and it is used by people of many different religions. Just like meditation or positive affirmations it is a way to bring balance into your life with the added benefit of healing your energy fields so that your body is healed as well.

Reiki does not infringe upon any religion and you may need to explain this to those who are asking for your help because if they feel as if they are doing something wrong the Reiki energy will focus on correcting the way they feel and not balancing out what is really wrong.

There are also those who believe if they use Reiki they are opening themselves up to psychic abilities or communication with the other side. This is because back in the 80's there was a book written by a woman who claimed that her students began seeing their spirit guide after using Reiki. Reiki is not going to give you any psychic abilities nor is it going to open you up to communicating with the other side, it is simply an exchange of healing energy.

Reiki is not a form of massage therapy. There are massage therapists that will offer Reiki sessions to their clients but Reiki does not involve any manipulation of bones or tissue. In fact you don't have to touch your clients when you are using Reiki, you can simply hover your hands above the person.

I also want you to understand that Reiki does not deplete the energy of the practitioner. Many people have believed this for a long time but the fact is that when you are a practitioner of Reiki, you are just channeling the energy, it is not your personal energy that is being used. If a person who is using Reiki feels tired after they have worked with a client it is usually because something is out of balance within themselves which is one more reason to make sure you are doing your daily self Reiki.

Once you have tuned in to Reiki, you may begin having a sense of peace and calmness, you may feel strangely positive, and may even start to have very vivid dreams. It is okay if you do not feel anything different right away this will come with time. When you begin feeling a change in your life you know you are ready to help others.

Before I begin explaining how really simple it is to help others by using Reiki, I want to talk a little bit about opening a practice. Many people once they begin being able to help those around them decide to open a Reiki practice in their home or outside of their home. While the purpose of using Reiki is not about making money it is understandable that you would want to charge a fee for your time.

What I want to make sure you understand is that you need to make sure you are actually helping people before you start charging an hourly rate for your services. Practice on yourself of course but also practice on your children or your friends. No harm will come to anyone who uses Reiki so you do not have to worry about getting it wrong. What you do need to worry about is giving people a false sense of hope when they come to you. If you do not have enough experience you will literally be taking their money and not providing them with any service.

Now on to helping those around you. Like I said I want you to practice self Reiki for at least 3 to 4 months and then you can begin practicing on your friends and family.

Reiki is actually very simple and I know it may seem complicated when you first begin but it really is not. Once you practice for a little while when you lay your hands on someone or something with the intent to heal them the energy will naturally flow through you. This really should take no effort on the part of the practitioner.

You do not have to perform any elaborate ritual when you begin a Reiki session, although some to bring their hands to their heart and bow in reverence to Reiki and asking Reiki to flow through them. You do not have to ask for Reiki to flow through you but it is out of respect that some do this.

When you begin using Reiki on someone you should not promise them specific results. As I said earlier Reiki goes where it is needed most and often this is very unpredictable. Instead tell your clients that Reiki will help them in the way that will benefit them the most because after all that is the truth.

When you place your hands on or above the person you are working with, it is not uncommon for the both of you to feel hot or cold sensations, vibrations, or tingling. Often times when the practitioner is feeling the sensation of heat, the receiver will feel a cold sensation so do not worry if your client is experiencing the opposite of what you are.

There are also times when the receiver will not feel a sensation in the moment but will feel it later in the day or even a few days later. And there will also be times when the receiver will feel no sensations at all but neither of you should worry because as long as you have put in the time to practice you can rest assured that Reiki is benefiting the client.

Chapter 12: Understanding Auras And How They Are Affected By Reiki

Processing energy isn't something that you are practicing consciously. It happens through us in ways that are not obvious, or always easily detectable. When you are learning about Reiki energy and the transformations that can occur as a result of shifting, purging and rebalancing energy systems, it might not seem like a lot is happening on the surface and it can take weeks and sometimes months for purges to actually open up the chakras for a better flow. It isn't always an instant gratification experience, especially when there could be decades of poor energy locked in your centers without any prior clearing or balancing.

All of the examples of how Reiki has allowed people to heal and live their lives in higher, more joyful and healthier ways are from those who have worked hard to learn from Reiki and use it as a tool on a regular, or daily basis. Energy purging and balancing can require daily tending with as little as some simple meditations or re-grounding. Besides just looking at how your chakras might be influenced by emotions and other experiences and stimuli, the auras are also subject to receiving and holding onto all kinds of energetic input from the world around, as well as projecting a similar kind of energy out into the world from within.

Have you ever stood in line next to someone at the bank and you could just feel how sad they were, without even seeing their eyes or face? Have you ever walked into a room and sensed that there was something really awkward and uncomfortable that just occurred? Those kinds of situations are all energetic and we are all always picking up and noticing those energetic imprints, whether we are fully conscious of it or not. There are plenty of ways that this kind of reality can manifest for an individual, but first let's break it down a little more so that you can understand the auric system and how it is related to the way we work with energetic transformations.

You Are an Energy Filter

Auras are not complicated; they are as simple as ABC and 123. You are always experiencing your life with your auras right out in front of you, first in line. There are already so many people today who have looked at pictures of their own aura readings from the technology that is able to capture it on film. This kind of a "energy report" is so exciting to see as it is a picture of proof that you are color and light. You are not able to see your chakras in this way, or any other reality of your internal make-up, without an x-ray or an MRI scan, and so to see something like the colorful light that emanates from your body is so exciting.

All of us have this light projection and it is called the auric field. The auras are a part of your chakras and are listening to everything going on inside and outside of you. They are the filter for what comes in and what goes out. You can ask someone if they are feeling okay, and they can tell you yes, but you are sure there is something else going on because you are picking up on another vibe from them. That is their auric field communicating with yours. All of us can do this, sense some else's auric field and energy, but so many people are not in awareness of it, or try to understand it because of their own focus on other realities of life.

You can be sure that the auras you are picking up on are full of junk that needs to be cleared, as there isn't a person alive today who is fully pure of all low vibration or negativity. People certainly get close and others are incredibly skilled and gifted at quickly releasing any input that wants to pass through their personal filtration system.

Let's use an example to make it clear: you just got off of work and are trying to get your dinner made so you can sit down and have a relaxing evening. You are in great spirits and feeling satisfied until your next-door neighbor rings the bell. You get up to answer and as you open the door you can feel a sudden change in your attitude and state of relaxation. Your neighbor is always at odds with another neighbor and has come over to gossip about them on your porch, just to satisfy their own energetic needs and problems.

You are picking up on all of their animosity and only allow a moment to pass before letting that person know that you are in the middle of your supper and would be happy to chat another time. When you return to your beautiful dinner at the table, you are no longer feeling satisfied and peaceful; you are now feeling unhappy and discombobulated after your encounter and are having a hard time returning to that delightful state of calm.

Your auric field was the first thing to answer the door and the other person's auric field was the first energy to greet you. You were not able to fully block their energy because you weren't expecting the visit and so your "filtrations system" was responsible for receiving the input and energy of the gossipy neighbor in just under a few minutes of conversation.

So, if you are in any situation with negative, or low feelings, you are likely picking up on all of that energy and taking it with you on some level. You may not even know that you are doing it and you will either unconsciously process it through other feelings and rebalance yourself naturally, or you may consciously notice the shift in your energy and clear it intentionally through some form of grounding and centering (Reiki, meditation, breathing, music, crystals, etc.).

If you are not able to recognize the energy exchange, or why you are suddenly feeling "off", you could end up travelling around with this energy as well as feeling something that isn't really yours to deal with and then have "stuck" or stagnate light in your auric field that needs to be purged. It's like going on a detox diet, but for energy.

Again, so much of this remains to be an unconscious experience for so many people, and even when people are well-informed about chakras and auras and how they work, we can still forget that other people's energy will influence us all day long. Not everyone is as energetically sensitive to these moments and experiences, and while some of us can see it come from a mile away, others are always looking at other methods of understanding their feelings, through therapy, counselling, doctor visits, etc., to pursue the answers to their "issues".

You are a filter for energy and you are also a projection of it. The next section explores the other side of energy, and how when it comes from within you and out toward the world and the people in it, it looks more like a projection.

You Are an Energy Projector

You have been to see a movie in a movie theater before; at least, I hope you have. Movies are images projected with light onto a screen so that we can see them. When you are living your life, you are projecting the energy of yourself into your auric field and out in to the screen of life to be received by everything around you at all times. It won't look like images on a movie screen, but it will perform to the reality of what you are exposing to the Universe through your auric field of light.

Our energy, be it emotional, mental, physical, or spiritual, will project itself outward through our chakras and eventually our auras until we are sharing our internal dance with the outside world. If you lack self-confidence and feel a need to overcompensate in some way by acting overly confident and egotistical, then you are projecting energy through your auras. If you are feeling like you are not as happy as everyone wants you to act so you try really hard to put on a smile and behave in accordance to what they suggest you do, then you are projecting an energy through your auras.

You can also project the energy of your highest vibration and joyful balance and harmony, but with these types of projections it is less of an actively unconscious pretense, and more of a radiation of higher vibrational energy that requires no projection; it just is. The goal of working with your energy is to get to a point where you don't have to project and you can just radiate higher vibrational energy.

When you are in alignment with your energy on a regular basis, you will find more opening and opportunity to radiate instead of project and it will become easier to notice when you are not in a balance with your highest vibration so that you can make necessary changes to balance yourself again.

Reiki, of course, is one of the most powerful ways to do this and when you are working with Reiki, you are working directly with the auric field and the chakra system.

The Anatomy of the Auric Field

The auras emanate from the skin layer, outward about 18 inches to 2 feet, give or take depending on the person and their personal energy. Each layer of your auric field is connected to one of the seven chakras. The chakras, as you learned in the last chapter, go from the root at the base of the spine to the crown of the head. From the deepest layer of your auric field, closest to your epidermis, you are connected to the root chakra energy. As you work your way out from the skin, you go through the layers of the chakras until you reach the crown layer, which will be the one farthest away from your body.

When you are looking at a picture of someone's aura and you only see one color, you are looking at the energy that is strongest in their auric field and as a result of that, how they are projecting their energy into the world. Other issues with the auric field that might come up for question is whether or not someone's auras can change color and the answer is, yes, they absolutely do. All of the time! When you are shifting and changing your energy frequency, either through intentional energy work, or through reality and life experience, your aura will change with you. It is like an aurora borealis and it isn't just a coincidence that the name of this gaseous light show in the arctic circle, and our auric field, have similar sounding names. In fact, the auras and the aurora borealis share similar qualities, as far as how quickly they can move from color to color through light, like waves on water under the moon.

There are plenty of studies today that are looking more deeply into the nature of our auras and how well they provide us with certain feedback and input for survival, intuition and instinct. There is a lot the science community has yet to prove or discover about the nature of the auric field, but in Reiki, it is one of the major components of healing work and the only proof necessary comes from trusting Reiki and FEELING with your own hands and energy what it is to touch the energy of another person.

Reiki and the Auric Field

When you are performing Reiki as a tool for energetic healing, you will be using the auric field to gauge the levels of need in the person who you are working on. There is a sense of this kind of energy read-out when you "comb" the aura with your hands. This appears as if you are holding your hand 4-12 inches, or so, above the body of the person who is receiving the

Reiki. When you comb the auric field, you are feeling the field with your hand chakras for any energetic input to give you guidance on where Reiki is most needed. It will look like you are waving the air around the outside of the client's body.

Part of the work that you do with the Reiki reading is that you will also find the tools that you need to work through the auric field on the chakras. You cannot effectively touch or reach the chakras from the outside of the body, but you can connect with the chakras through the auric field and what each layer of aura represents on the outside of the body. Therefore, working through the auric field is like working on the chakras themselves.

You can learn these tools and techniques later in the book and while you are asking more questions about the auric field and the chakras in your Reiki work, they will teach you everything you need to know as you go through the channeling and healing process. You will be amazed at the kinds of assessment you can do with Reiki as your guide. It is a very intuitive experience and the more you practice "reading" and "combing" the auras and energy, the more you will understand just how it works and what it is there to show you.

Now that you have a deeper knowledge of the auric field and Reiki, we can move to the next chapter to go over what Reiki really is and exactly how it works. The information from the first four chapters has set you up to fully understand why Reiki works and how it can be such a powerful tool for healing.

Chapter 13: Attributes Of A Reiki Master

I believe if you are reading this book you aim to be a Reiki Master someday. Before we get into Reiki healing practices, there are few things you should know. Reiki is guided by the divine, this means that if you are controlled by the flesh you may never obtain that Master status.

Mikao Usui's guidelines for living which was part of his entire life was the awareness that you are meant to serve with this tremendous power. You have to be spiritually awakened and control the urges of the flesh. I will deal with three personality traits that once eradicated, would take you to the highest level of your Reiki mastering.

Anger and Worry

It is natural to get angry and by no means do I mean you should suppress your anger. To become a Reiki master, don't get yourself wound up in things of no importance. Put everything in its proper perspective. You have to learn to let go of hurts, disappointments, and pain and understand that people are fundamentally limited. Don't worry about the things you cannot change, this drains out energy from you and you won't be in control of your own mind.

Humility

You have to understand that you're a channel through which the divine flows, do not act like you have all the answers. If you ever want to be a master, don't let the miracles you see get into your head. Remind yourself constantly that you're a source of hope and joy and you have to stay humble to keep doing the good work. Also, look around you at the things that give you so much joy, be thankful for that and be grateful.

Compassion

This is very vital if you want to become a Reiki Master. This applies to you as much as you are to others. Care for yourself, care for others. If you don't take care of yourself, you won't do a proper job. Understand that people depend on you sometimes as their final hope and to do an effective job, you have to feel their pain and be in a mindful state to heal them.

Honesty

You have to be honest with yourself and be honest in the way you treat people to become a true Reiki Master. What are your motives for learning Reiki? Are they true and honest? Do they benefit just you and your own ambitions? Reiki isn't meant to encourage selfishness. You have to remember that Reiki is not all about you, you have to be honest about this to those who attend your classes or your healing sessions.

Chapter 14: Reiki And Meditation

Meditation is a common practice in Reiki. Many holistic healers and practitioners do include meditation of some kind in their lives. Whether they are yoga instructors, massage therapists, Reiki practitioners, or individuals that are committed to a full body, mind, and spirit wellness will use meditation regularly.

There are two basic forms of meditation. The first is to completely clear your mind of all thoughts. The second type of meditation is to focus on a specific question, concern, or situation.

With Reiki meditation, the focus is on Reiki energy rather than any other subject. During a Reiki meditation, you focus on the universal energy as it is within you, around you, and within everything around you. You want to feel connected to that energy to create a feeling of tranquility, connection, and peace.

Your body will feel revitalized and full of life energy. It is a very rejuvenating type of meditation.

When you meditate, it is recommended that you find a quiet place where you won't be disturbed. You'll want to set a relaxing atmosphere. Set the lights low, light some candles, maybe burn some incense or diffuse herbal oils. If music helps you relax, play a soothing soundtrack.

You can sit or lie down for meditation, but if you are prone to falling asleep, sitting up may be the best idea. While it isn't bad to fall asleep during meditation, the goal is to keep a certain focus and connection with the Reiki energy which won't be as strong if you fall asleep.

To start relaxing your mind, breathe in through your nose to the count of four and then breathe out through your mouth to the count of eight.

After a few of these deep breaths, you'll want to start focusing on Reiki energy. Start with the energy within yourself, and as you connect to it, feel it expand outward into the universe and into the space and objects around you. You should feel the energy moving through you and around you.

Keep your focus on that energy for as long as you want to, or as long as you feel called to. If you want to meditate for a certain amount of time, set some kind of timer with a gentle call back sound like a soft bell or gong to let you when you should end the meditation.

Meditation can take practice. If you are unfamiliar with meditation or new to meditation, you might have to work your way up to longer meditation times. Starting with just five minutes is fairly standard.

In the beginning, it is easy to get distracted by thoughts and sounds in the room around you, like the heat coming on, the sound of a branch on the window, or thoughts of your day. Over time, with practice, these distractions won't be as prominent.

However, there are some techniques to help you stay in that meditative mindset.

One method to try is when you begin to meditate, set the tip of your tongue to the top of your mouth. If your mind starts to wander, your tongue will fall from the roof of your mouth. Any time you notice this, bring your tongue back to the roof of your mouth and refocus on your meditation.

The tongue trick is somewhat similar to the Gassho finger technique in which you press your middle fingers together if you begin to experience thoughts that pull you away from your meditation. Starting a meditation with the Gassho technique can also help your mind focus when you move into a Reiki meditation.

There is a somewhat standard 21-day Reiki meditation program that can help you learn more about Reiki and also help you develop your meditation skills. It is broken down into different segments to cover the 21 days. These 21 days are also symbolic of the time that Dr. Usui spent on top of a mountain in study to reach enlightenment.

Chapter 15: The Third Eye And Reiki

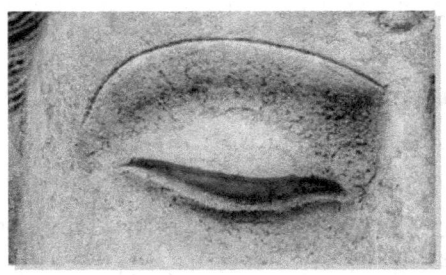

Your third eye chakra is between your eyes and it deals with intelligence and psychic power. The colors associated with the third eye are violet, deep blue, and indigo.

As you perhaps know from biology, *hormones* are responsible for how the body functions. Hormones are tied to many aspects of your body including the physical, emotional, and mental aspects. Modern day Reiki practitioners relate chakras to the *endocrine system*.

Functions of the Third Eye Chakra

For your physical health, the third eye governs the pineal gland along with your eyes, ears, nose, and the skeletal system. It is tied to the senses of sight and hearing as well as one's ability to form their own opinions about the world around them and how they are going to live.

Your third eye secretes a hormone known as *melatonin* which regulates your sleep cycle and growth and also slows down the aging process while maintaining a stable mind. This gland is sensitive to light which makes most people believe that the eyes are stimulated from the pineal gland when melatonin is released. Many scientists think that the electromagnetic field of the earth is also responsible for stimulating this gland.

Your pineal gland governs your eyes and how you see the world around you, as well as any psychic and intuitive abilities you may have.

The third eye chakra plays a vital role in determining how alert you will be, as well as help with how clearly you see things and how optimistic you are while you visualize the outcomes you want. This chakra will create a reality for you that can become real based on your perception. Whenever this chakra is balanced, you will have the ability to visualize better and your memory will become sharper. You should trust yourself that you can be able to rely on your intuitions. You will also be able to help someone without them requesting for your help.

An imbalanced third eye chakra causes problems in understanding reality or creating our own. You may find that you are relying too much on luck and blaming someone when a bad situation happens. Your headache will cause trouble on you which will also lead to having a constant feeling of anxiousness. You may find that you want to dominate or control others. If you experience these things, then your third eye is blocked.

Using Reiki to Unblock Your Third Eye

Reiki practitioners have their own methods of working the third eye chakra. However most often the following basic steps are used to help you clear your third eye chakra with Reiki:

Chapter 16: What Is Community-Based Reiki?

Good question. Now I guess I have to find a succinct answer, don't I? Community-Based Reiki is a framework that will let you design a targeted outreach program to reach a chosen population in an efficient and effective manner for the purpose of….oh dear, too much jargon? I thought so.

I'll do my best to keep the jargon to a minimum, but it won't be easy. I loved working in Health Education and I miss it very much. For the past few years I've been working in a professional healthcare office and it's not nearly as much fun as creatively impacting lives through Health Education.

Health Education is a social science that blends all kinds of science—biological, environmental, psychological, medical—to promote health and wellness through education and other voluntary behavior change activities. Preventing disease, disability, and premature death is all part of the Health Education ball of wax.

Writing this book is like coming home for me. These terms and concepts are old friends. They say you should "write what you know". Well, I know this stuff. It's a blend of Health Education, Behavior Modification, Community Organizing, and Sociology. If I can avoid the jargon and keep you awake, you'll know this stuff, too, and by the end of the book you'll be able to use it. It's easier than you think to turn your ideas into tangible results.

But I'm getting ahead of myself. What were you asking? Oh, yes. What is Community-Based Reiki?

Community-Based Reiki is a framework that helps you and the other Reiki Practitioners in your area work together to take the Reiki things you like to do—and the Reiki things you **wish** you could do—and turn them into something amazing that gets Reiki to more people than you ever thought possible.

Typically, people look at Reiki through a Medical Model, where you work with one individual at a time to address symptoms and problems for people who are already ill. Community-based Reiki operates from a Public Health standpoint. Here, the community, itself, is the patient and improving the health of the population is the goal. Disease prevention and health promotion take place through organized efforts that work with groups of people, as well as with individuals.

In a Public Health program, professionals review the health of a population and diagnose its problems. Then they look for the causes of those problems and come up with strategies to address them. The Public Health approach works along with the Medical Model to improve the health of the community, exactly like Reiki works in cooperation with traditional medicine to bring healing to your asthmatic brother.

It's not a case of either/or, but a time to work together for the best possible outcome for the patient, whether your patient is a horse, your 5th cousin, or everyone in your zip code with juvenile diabetes.

There have probably been plenty of times when you wished you could do more to make your community healthier, you just didn't know how to do it. Community Reiki won't tell you exactly what to do; instead it will help you figure that out for yourself.

You see, you and the other Reiki Practitioners in your town are the experts when it comes to expanding Reiki in your area. How could an outsider tell you what to do? You are custom-made for your time and your place. Reiki works with you and through you in a way that no one else can match.

This isn't some kind of cookie cutter approach where "One Size Fits All" for every one in every city in every country. You'll design your own local Community Reiki outreach. This way it will be perfectly suited to you and the unique opportunities and challenges of your particular community. Community Reiki is one of those "grow where you're planted" concepts where the actions you take are based on the realities of where you are.

Besides, you have a distinct advantage over me and my old Health Education cronies from "back in the day" when we worked to reduce smoking in California: You don't have to write up a giant 300-page Progress Report for the State on your activities and send the original plus five copies of it up to Sacramento to be reviewed and critiqued like I did…..twice a year. Ah! Good Times.

What you do have is Reiki energy on your side and all of the extra tools it brings into play. Got a tough choice to make? Meditate, use a pendulum, or do some Byosen Scanning over each option to feel which one has the best energy.

How Do I Use This Book?

At its most basic level, you can use this book as a paperweight, or maybe to even out a tippy table by shoving it under the short leg, but if you're reading this as an e-book, I wouldn't recommend that. It would be a pretty serious thing to hold up a table with your entire library. And about that paperweight suggestion? In a few more years I wouldn't be surprised if someone read that and asked "What is this thing you call 'paper'?" Yes, the times they are a-changing.

Let me repeat: The times they are a-changing. And you're going to help them a-change. Where this book inspires you, follow that passion. If some ideas in this book intimidate or bore you, pull back and stick with the concepts that are a better fit. This is a handbook you can refer to again and again. Whatever step you take now is the right step for you. It doesn't have to be a big step for man or a giant leap for mankind. Big or small, every bit of Reiki you put out there helps the world move forward in love and light.

As you read, you're going to be exposed to some new ideas for using Reiki. It may take a while for those ideas to simmer before you can chew on them. In time, you'll be ready to take a few more bites.

Or maybe not. That's OK. Universal Life Energy works in mysterious ways. So read on, take what you can use, and put the rest into storage.

What Exactly Am I Going to be Learning?

You would ask that, wouldn't you?

Let me guess. Toastmasters. You've been in Toastmasters, right? The group that helps people develop public speaking abilities. Yeah. I've never been to one of their meetings, but I know one of the big ideas they hammer home is this: Tell the audience what you're going to tell them, tell it to them, and then tell them what you told them.

It's a good way to frame a speech or public presentation. It's also a good way to introduce a handbook that is a basic manual to help you accomplish something. I've been a little evasive so far, haven't I? "Help you accomplish something". Is that really what I said? This book is a manual that will "help you accomplish something". What? How?? For whom???

EXACTLY!!!!!!

You've hit on it perfectly! This book will help you figure out "what" and "how" and "who". WHAT you're going to do. HOW you're going to do it. WHO you're going to target. You'll learn how to work together with other Reiki Practitioners in your area, how to narrow your focus for greater impact where Reiki healing is needed the most, and how to effectively create lasting change.

I've heard more than one story of a person who prepared to do some serious Reiki healing after receiving their Reiki training. They had the "If You Build It, They Will Come" vibe and ordered their Reiki table, printed up some business cards, and rented a space. Then they sat, wondering where all the clients were. Many of the techniques in this manual can be used to help you build your practice.

My main intent, though, is to help you form a team of local Reiki Practitioners so you can work with others to expand the use of Reiki in your community, getting healing energy out where it is needed the most. This will help bring greater health and wellness to the people who live around you, healing your corner of the world. It will also automatically create more demand for all Reiki services in your area.

Soooooo...first this book will walk you through the things you can do to build your Reiki Team. Then it's going to help you and your Reiki Team go through the steps to figure out how to expand Reiki in your area so it reaches and teaches others who need Reiki and are ready for it. This book is going to help you get that Reiki canoe over to people so they can hop on when they are good and ready to jump off that roof and move into uncharted waters.

But wait! There's more! These pages are going to help you take your goal and break it down into simple activities to make your goal a reality. Then you're going to hop up to the advanced level and learn some ways to evaluate those activities so you can know if you're really making a difference. And THEN, you are going to learn how to write mini-grants to get funding for your projects.

Yes. For the ideas you have. For the plan you made up. For the activities you created out of thin air. Yes, all that stuff you and your local Reiki Team imagined into being. You are going to learn the basics of how to write mini-grants to gain funding so you can accomplish more than you ever thought possible. Don't be afraid to dream big! After all, you're not doing this all on your own.

There! I've followed the Toastmasters model: I told you what I'm going to tell you. Whew! That's a lot for one book! But I'll make you a deal: We'll get through it together. I'm here with you every step of the way. We'll take baby steps. You and me. Working together.

Well, look at that! We just created our very own Reiki Team! See how easy that was?

Chapter 17: My Introduction To Reiki

I had a vague notion that Reiki was some kind of relaxing technique, but that's all I knew until I experienced it. My world changed when I stepped through the front door of a single wide mobile home in northwest New Mexico and found myself in a living room that was the work space for a Reiki practitioner.

When my massage therapist suggested I go to this woman, I didn't realize she was not only a Reiki Master but also a medicine woman, who had discovered her healing abilities as a child. Short in stature with long hair, a smiling face and tattoos on her arm, she welcomed me into her Reiki room. It contained a massage table, feathers, rattles, tuning forks, ear cones, live plants, a water fall, and an assortment of other tools. Without preamble, she told me to lie on the table. I heard rattles, felt feathers and soon fell into a restful state deeper than sleep.

When the session ended, I felt so refreshed that I wanted to experience more. After several treatments, she suggested that I could give Reiki to myself if I received the Reiki I attunement in a special one-on-one ceremony.

Because I loved the way Reiki made me feel, I agreed to move forward even though I wasn't sure what an attunement was. She told me to read *Essential Reiki: A Complete Guide to an Ancient Healing Art* by Diane Stein. I bought the book, and read it as well as *Reiki, the Healing Touch: First and Second Degree Manual* by William Lee Rand. Armed with a better understand of what I was getting into, I called her to schedule the attunement.

The ceremony took less than half an hour. I sat on a piano stool with my eyes closed and followed her directions as she moved around me, drawing in my hands and doing something above my head and down my back. When the ceremony ended, I began to cry. Something had opened and expanded in me.

"This is not new to you," she said. "You have been a Reiki healer before. Your guides are so happy you have chosen this pathway again."

That felt right, even though my conservative Christian background didn't recognize guides or past lives.

For about a week after the attunement, my body buzzed with so much energy I felt like I'd stuck my finger in a light socket. I discovered that touching trees helped ease the overcharged energy. Trees willingly took some of it from me.

I gave myself Reiki every day for a month and a half before I scheduled a Reiki II attunement, which took me deeper into the healing method. I began to practice on friends, and their responses increased my confidence. They told me that they found relief from pain or discovered better ways to handle personal relationships and challenging events.

I wanted to learn more so I could teach Reiki and practice it on an even deeper level. Six months later, I received the Reiki Master attunement from the medicine woman. Her method didn't include much teaching, so I read everything I could about Reiki.

For a year and a half I gave free Reiki sessions at a local community college to introduce Reiki to others and to give myself practice. Then I began working with other professionals at a local alternative healing clinic.

A year after receiving my Reiki Master attunement, I taught Reiki to someone else and passed the Reiki I attunement to them. Since then, I've taught other workshops and passed Reiki I, Reiki II and Reiki Master attunements to other students.

My practice doesn't involve feathers, tuning forks, and rattles. My tools are simpler — a Reiki table, prayer, and sometimes a few crystals, which help to focus or intensify the healing energy. The more experience I have with Reiki and the more I learn about it from other gifted healers and writers, I have come to understand certain things about this amazing healing art.

Reiki, which flows with the light of unconditional love, draws people into a place of deep rest and relaxation. In this place, it's easier for the body's incredible healing abilities to work.

Reiki is a Japanese word, which means spiritually guided universal life energy. The word *rei* describes universal, higher knowledge, or spiritual consciousness, while the word *ki* refers to the non-physical energy in all living things.

Though giving and receiving Reiki is a spiritual experience, it is not a religion. It's a healing art. You don't have to adopt any set of beliefs to practice it. You don't even have to believe that Reiki will work. It works whether you think it will or not.

A healer's hands help to guide the flow of Reiki energy. Some people follow a set pattern of hand positions. Others intuitively sense where to place their hands.

During the healing session, a connection forms between those who give and receive Reiki. They both benefit from it. So do many others, because Reiki spreads far beyond your physical location. It goes for miles, benefitting anyone who is willing to receive it. When you practice Reiki, you share unconditional love with countless others you may never meet.

The symbol for Reiki helps to explain the healing practice. The first character, *rei*, shows that, just as plants need water for healthy growth, people flourish when they combine prayer and work. Raindrops are pictured as four lines within a cloud. Three squares represent mouths open in prayer. A reclining H, which looks like an early farm tool to prepare the ground for planting, shows the concept of work.

The *ki* character paints a picture of steam coming from cooked rice or of water vapor rising from the ground and turning into rain, which brings nourishment to plants. The earth nurtures plants, and the sky waters them, creating the energy of new life. *1*

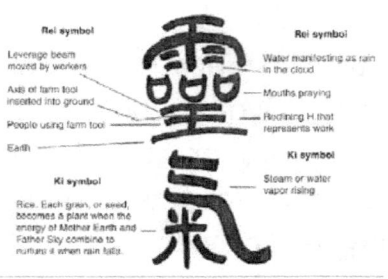

Reiki Symbol and Its Meaning

In a similar way, God directs the flow of Reiki energy. It travels through Reiki practitioners to those who need it, helping to sustain, nurture and heal them. If you feel uncomfortable with the word God, use whatever term you like to refer to the source of unconditional love, the creator of all that is.

Chapter 18: Angelic Reiki Basics Synopsis

Working hand in hand with the Angelic Realms, Ascended Master collective and Galactic Beings, Angelic Reiki provides a sound system of healing and consciousness expansion. It's a mighty means of personal growth, transformation and readying for ascending. It's the healing for our time.

Angelic Reiki is a mighty healing modality that works with the highest powers of the Angelic Realm to manifest healing and balance on all layers to those getting the healing power. With Angelic Reiki we have the chance for self healing and to send out healing to others, places and situations near and far away.

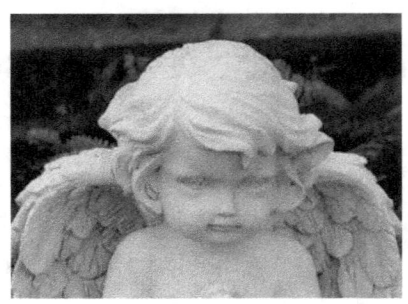

The Basics

Angelic Reiki uses disciplines from the Usui and Shamballa lineages and blends these with mighty transmissions channeled by masters.

This is a total system of energy healing which is open to all. The attunements ready and initiate people to begin working hand in hand with Angelic Beings of Light and found a conscious and lasting link with the Angelic Dimension.

During an Angelic Reiki treatment, the practician is merely a bridge for the angelic healing power to pass to the receiver.

Angels are not confined by time and space. Working in alignment and together with Angels and Archangels consequently helps us to reach deeply into all areas which call for rebalancing and healing. In multidimensional Angelic Reiki healing, the receiver is lovingly supported to relinquish physical, emotional and karmic imbalances as well as ancestral problems throughout all time and space. It's a blessing to give and get these angelic healing sessions.

The utilization of Angel Reiki has the same precepts as Usui Reiki.

Archangel Raphael is the angel of healing, although there are a lot more Angels and Archangels that will help you to heal yourself and or a set of circumstances. Angels have limitless healing powers and may heal emotional and physical pain. Simply ask for their help for your own personal healing.

The treatment of Angel Reiki is the same as Usui Reiki, hands off / on and remote healing. An individual might wish to remain sitting upright or laid on a couch, as with all reiki you remain totally clothed throughout the treatment session. The atmosphere is produced utilizing relaxing music, which may greatly benefit the treatment, likewise helping the person to relax quicker.

The Angel Reiki power is channeled from the angelic realm with the help of Ascended masters, Archangels and Angels, which is then passed through the hands of the healer to the individual wanting to receive healing.

Angels may help us to reach the realms that need to be readdressed, that call for balancing and healing, likewise allowing you to be lovingly supported to relinquish physical, emotional and karmic imbalances.

The utilization of crystals may also be used to help remove and heal blocks.
Angel Reiki is soft and loving.

All Reiki is the procedure of working with a person's energy system. The aim is to get rid of unwanted damaging energy and replace it with harmonious, favorable and healthy energy.

Chapter 19: A Typical Usui Reiki Session

Although the Usui School is the original, it is not unified since the founder did teach thousands of pupils who have put their own slant on his teachings and practices. The following is therefore a basic standard for those who follow the Usui method.

Wear loose, comfortable clothing for a session. Before it proceeds, you will be asked to remove all jewelry, including watches, as well as anything made of metal. It's believed that metal interferes with the flow of energy. If you have metal braces that can't be removed, let the practitioner know so they can work around it.

According to adherents, the energy is an intelligent one, so it can adapt itself according to the recipient's needs. This means that reiki can also be performed by and on pregnant women.

Your practitioner will wash his/her hands in cold water and may perform certain hand movements around the room before working on you. This is to energize the space and clear it of any negative energies. Washing also ensures that they are free of negative energy and that they don't carry anything from a previous session onto yours. When the session is completed, they will wash their hands again.

If you are given a bed or massage table to lie on, you will be asked to keep your legs straight and not to cross them. You will also lay your arms by your sides, but not cross them over your chest or stomach. Your head will also be elevated by a pillow. The practitioner will cover your body with a blanket or large towel, but leave your face uncovered. There is to be no talking during a session, unless you need to communicate something very important.

They'll then stand at your head, raise their arms on either side with their palms up and say: "I offer (your name) love and healing through the universal life force energy," or use some other similar wording.

They will then place their hands over or touch the twelve parts of your body cited earlier. They will also cover your legs and feet.

Once your session is over, you will be left alone for a few minutes to give you time to recover naturally and as relaxed as possible. It is customary to have an after-session talk with the practitioner to discuss any concerns you may have or to plan a future session.

If you've had at least one session with a practitioner, but can't make it to another one, they can perform it without you. This is called distance reiki or reiki in absentia. This can only be done by a qualified reiki practitioner, however, and only by one who has already had contact with you. It's believed that those who've already made a connection with you can transmit the ki regardless of distance. In such cases, you must be in a relaxed state and be aware that the session is going on to best receive that energy.

Chapter 20: About Chakras Including The Third Eye

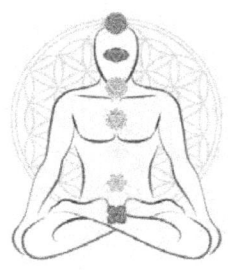

What is chakra?
A Chakra (pronounced "cha"-"kra") is a center of energy. The word chakra comes from Sanskrit (a religious language of India), and its name literally means "wheel" because of its vortex of energy. It spins and interacts with many different physiological and neurological systems in the body. Chakras or "energy centers," help to regulate all of the processes from a person's emotions to their organ functions, including the body's immune system.

There are twelve chakras; seven primary and five secondary. These chakras fall into two types of configurations. They are all either located inside of the body, or they are both inside and outside of the body. In modern schools of thought, the primary chakras are located inside of the body while the additional chakras are located on the outside.

It is important to learn and understand each of their individual energies and the connection they have to our universe. This powerful system works to balance our energies. When restoring the power of chakras, it will give you control over your health and well-being.

Since Reiki was rediscovered, its energy flow has been used to effect the way energy moves throughout the body. Reiki was primarily used to concentrate on one energy center that is located in the lower abdomen area, but there are actually three areas in total. The other two are in the upper chest and in the center of the forehead.

Chakra healing originates from a Hindu practice and has also played an important part in Buddhism. The energy healing from chakras involves the focus of energy healing from points in the body, from under the feet to above the head. These points are called "meridians," or energy lines that flow through and outside of the body. They are all points responsible for regulating energy flow.

About the Chakras

Hinduism teaches that the body's natural reservoir of energy automatically pools at several different points throughout the body. Each of these points acts as a type of nexus between the physical body and what is known as the subtle body. Each of the points on the subtle body then interacts directly with one of many different subtle planes of existence. When these all come together, they combine to create the physical world we are more directly familiar with. Each one of these planes connect directly to a different state of consciousness, outside of the one where you likely spend the majority of your time. These states of consciousness include ego, mind, and intelligence which all combine to control the physical body.

In addition, each of the chakras can also be thought of as an energy portal that connects to all the rest through specific Nadi, or energy channels, that run throughout the subtle body. All told, there are seven primary chakras spread throughout the body. They are:

Sahasrara: This chakra is most frequently known as the crown chakra and is primarily associated with a state of pure consciousness wherein both subjects and objects cease to exist in their present form. When your natural energy is extremely high, it can combine with the male Shiva energy that resides in the crown chakra and form a state of meditative consciousness like no other. This state is known as Samadhi, and it is prized above all other meditative states. The crown chakra is frequently represented as a lotus flower with 1,000 differing petals, each a unique color. It can be found at the very top of the head and is often represented by pure whiteness. It is effective when called upon to deal with extreme hardship, things like the death of the mortal body and the search for true enlightenment.

Ajna: More commonly known as the third eye, Ajna is also the "mind's eye" or "inner eye". It is a mystical and cryptic concept of an abstract, invisible eye which gives perception beyond normal sight.

The third eye chakra is located in the center of the forehead between both eyes and oversees the intelligence and psychic power according to Hindu tradition.

Hindu healers referred to this principle as Ajna and it is often symbolized by the OM symbol, with a flower petal on each side. The associated colors are deep blue, indigo and sometimes the color, violet.

The point where it is located is said to be the point where the Nadi Pingala and the Nadi Ida merge with the primary Sushuma Nadi channel, putting to rest the duality of their existence. The main deity associated with this chakra is Ardhanarishvara, a being known to be both male and female.

It is often associated with the third eye's ability to see outside the prime material plane and can be invoked when additional guidance and balance are needed or when you need a boost to your intuition.

The third eye chakra controls the pineal gland, eyes, ears, nose, and the skeletal system. It is related to the senses of sight and hearing and has the ability to know and understand in order to form opinions about what is seen and how it exists.

The pineal gland's main role is to secrete a hormone called, "melatonin," which plays a part in regulating sleep patterns, growth, slowing down aging, and also maintaining a stable mind. This pineal gland is sensitive to light, that is the reason the eyes stimulate the pineal gland by releasing the melatonin. It was discovered that the earth's electromagnetic field is responsible for stimulating the gland as well.

The third eye chakra is important to be able to see things clearly and not just physically. Its role is in making you see things clearly, not only physically, but morally and intuitively.

This chakra also plays a role in governing awareness, as well as the way you see and predict things to visualize the desired positive outcomes. This chakra is responsible for the ability to form perceptions about reality. When in balance, this chakra will help you easily and clearly visualize memory and reason. You will begin to trust your judgment and intuitions. An imbalance, however, can cause reality misunderstanding, causing you to rely too much on fate if something negative happens. Trouble in the form of headaches and a feeling of anxiousness, worry, and control issues will result as well. Every one of these is a sign that there is a blocked third eye chakra.

Practice love and tolerance to unblock this chakra. Giving yourself recognition for the things that you accomplish; especially practicing self-love. By focusing positively on all things in your life and how much you have yet to accomplish you will help to rid yourself of many psychological and physical problems.

The practice of meridians and energy flow are the same in both Reiki and Chakra systems, but the fact that there are seven major chakras makes it easier to give specific Reiki treatment for physical health issues.

Vishuddha: More commonly known as the throat chakra, Vishuddha is frequently drawn as a silver crescent suspended inside a white circle and surrounded by blue petals, or possibly a red crescent with 16 upward facing petals instead. Vishuddha promotes lucid dreaming along with the communication and growth that occurs when a group of individuals gets together in order to fully express their feelings and thoughts. It is also frequently described as being one of the primary influences relating to security, spirituality, new ideas, and independence.

Anahata: More frequently referred to as the heart chakra, Anahata is typically represented as a round flower with green petals, called the heartmind, and is said to be the visual expression of humanity's need to be connected to other living things. Inside this flower is a pair of triangles that are positioned in such a way that they form a hexagram that represents the unity between male and female. This chakra is frequently discussed as being connected to the thymus which is a critical part of the immune and endocrine systems. It is generally connected to the colors pink and green along with the more complicated emotions related to personal well-being, tenderness, equilibrium, and unconditional love.

Manipura: This chakra is located between the naval and the solar plexus and is typically presented as a yellow triangle with 5 yellow leaves on each side. It is typically thought of as being associated with a well-functioning immune system and ensuring that the body can easily turn food into energy. It is always associated with the color yellow and is frequently used when it comes to dealing with the transition between strong opinions or emotions as well as feelings of fear, introversion, anxiety or the issues that arise with concerns over using the power of status correctly.

Svadhisthana: This chakra is more commonly known as the sacral chakra and it is located in the middle of the sacrum. It is most commonly associated with the ovaries as well as the testes and is known to help keep the body's sex hormones working properly and ensure the reproductive system functions as it should. It is most often called upon when it comes to dealing with emotions related to emotional desires like intimacy, violence, addiction, and pleasure.

Muladhara: More commonly referred to as the root chakra, Muladhara is most frequently drawn as a lotus with four red petals. It is located near the base of the spine and is connected to the adrenal medulla as well as the gonads. This chakra is commonly associated with security, sexuality, stability, and survival. It is also at this point that the main Nadi separates and moves upward towards the Sahasrara. This is also where the dormant kundalini energy in your body lies in wait, wrapped three and a half times around the first three obstructions that you will need to overcome if you ever hope to have a kundalini awakening.

Chakra healing also helps with spiritual and emotional treatment. Each of the seven chakras closely aligns with mental well-being. A Reiki practitioner can find a blockage or even where one had been if they have studied and are working with the emotional system within chakra healing; then they can apply energy to that area. A practitioner working with Reiki can be a huge benefit to chakra healing systems. Other things that will help include:

- Meditation
- Yoga
- Using chakra healing stones
- Eating foods or spices associated with a specific chakra
- Aromatherapy

If our life energy is balanced or flowing well, it is believed that our mental, emotional, physical, and spiritual well-being will be in a much better condition as a result. Reiki restores the balance of your energy flow if you are going through physical or emotional stress. Even though it is not a substitute for medical attention, it can work along with medical assistance to achieve things that medical science alone cannot. Also, Reiki can be offered to new parents and babies, people suffering from trauma, law enforcement, and individuals with mental health or addiction problems as well as with small and large corporate health programs.

Chakra balancing, opening chakras and using chakra techniques, should be instrumental when it comes to ensuring your well-being and overall health. Many health practices are using these guiding principles as a foundation to health systems and a sustainable flow of energy. These medical practices often begin with old or traditional principles of Eastern spirituality as well as modern healing techniques, that often began with these practices. Today's healing techniques have evolved through the years — thanks to people that come from a large range of energy healing and holistic medical fields. In modern time, healers relate chakras with the endocrine system of the body. This system releases hormones that regulate many actions including growth and development, changes, and functions.

Reiki practitioners each have ways to work with the third eye chakra. The following is one way to work with this process to clear you third eye chakra.

There are also many other methods to use. A mantra (steady use of repeated soft words or phrases) will aid in healing. The vibration radiating from the mantra will help to open the chakra energy forces. Use of aromatherapy can be helpful, especially mint and jasmine.

Chapter 21: Crystal Cleansing Techniques

Crystal healing and Reiki both are two different healing modalities and yet both goes together hand in hand. When Reiki andcrystals are combined for healing, the result is magnificent. Having crystals along while healing with Reiki energy is like having an extra pair of hands. Since learning Reiki, I have developed a great liking towards. I have to strictly stop myself from purchasing any and every crystal I come across. Some crystals resonates with me so well as if they are just meant for me. Just holding some crystals in palms starts vibration in third eye. Having bought lots of crystals, next thing is to take care of them. Cleansing crystal is the most important thing to do before a healing session, setting a grid or programming for any other use. Those who are new to crystals may start wondering why crystals need cleansing. I asked hubby to give me his crystal pendant to cleanse. He said, "no its ok, it is not dirty☐". Actually crystal tends to absorb the energies around them. To diffuse the accumulated negative energy, we need to cleanse crystal. Cleansing removes all the previous programming too. So once cleansed, charge and program your crystals. Let us explore few crystal cleansing methods here:-

Note- I would suggest to use reiki symbols and reiki flow for every cleansing method. Reiki all the cleansing material used- salt, water, container, candle etc

Salt Water- Add salt to water and soak crystals for few hours in salt water. Not all crystals resonates with salt and water, so check before soaking crystals.

Dry Salt- Place your crystals in a bowl of dry sea salt/rock salt/Himalayan salt. Make sure there are no left over salt particles once you are done cleansing.

Running water- Hold your crystal under a tap, stream or any form of fresh running water. Imagine all the accumulated negative energy flowing away with running water.

Earth- Place your crystals back to its original cradle. Bury your crystals in your garden, planter or backyard. Alternatively, gather some soil in a container and bury your crystal. After removing, wipe it clean and make sure no soil particles are left.

Breathe- Hold your crystal in your palm and blow forcefully on your crystal. Imagine you are blowing a white light over crystals. Keep blowing till you feel your crystal is shiny or simply blow thrice with the intention to cleanse.

Flame- Just rotate your crystal 7 times over a candle flame to cleanse it. You can even pass your crystal quickly through flame.

Moon/Sun- This is one of the simplest and safest method. Simply leave your crystals out in sunlight or moon light. Not all crystals resonates with sunlight so please check crystal's properties before placing in sunlight.

Smudging - Use sage or incense stick to cleanse the crystal. Simply pass your crystal through sage/incense stick smoke.

Reiki only- Hold crystal in palm and draw CKR, Give reiki with the intention to remove negative energy from the crystal.

Bell or Singing Bowl- The vibration of the bell or the singing bowl has the power to cleanse your crystals. Just play the sound of bell/singing bowl near the crystals.

Selenite- Selenite is considered as 'Universal Stone Cleaner'. It does not need cleansing. Simply place your crystal over a selenite cluster or place selenite over your crystal. Alternatively, put all crystals in a box and program your selenite to cleanse all crystals in the box.

Beach- Going to a beach? Take your crystal along and cleanse with sea water.

Pendulum- Program your pendulum to cleanse the crystal and hold it over your crystal.

Third Eye- Direct white light on your crystals with your third eye with the set intention.

Crystal Clusters/Geode- Some crystals (citrine, carnelian, selenite) doesn't need frequent cleansing. They can be used to cleanse other crystals too. Simply place your crystals on the geode or cluster.

Plants- Lay your crystal besides your favorite flower or plant. Plants has the natural ability to transmute negative energy to positive energy.

Pyramid dome- The shape of a pyramid itself is very powerful. Place your crystals under the pyramid dome. Pyramid dome neutralizes the accumulated negative energy of crystals when placed inside the dome.

Flower essence- Soak flower petals of any flower in water for few hours. Fill this water in a spray bottle and spray on crystals.

Again, for any of the above method, cleansing done with invoking symbols and infusing reiki will optimize cleansing, charging and programing.

Diseases and associated chakras

Here is an article especially written for new reiki practitioners. At one point in our reiki practice, many of us were in a dilemma about which chakra to heal for certain disease/problem. When I was a newbie in reiki, I always wondered about which chakra was to be healed for particular problem/disease. I used to browse through the internet for long hours to satisfy my queries. Many new reiki practitioners go through this same confusion. We read about chakras, their colors, crystal healing etc, yet for new practitioners it's quite confusing as to which chakra is associated with which disease. Recently I have gotten queries about which chakras are to be healed for certain problems. Hence I thought of making this list with a few common problems/disease and chakras associated with them, especially for new reiki practitioners. I am not writing about chakras and their functions. Below is just a list of diseases/problems and associated chakras.

CROWN
- Alzheimer,
- Amnesia, Bone disorders,
- Cancers,
- Depression,

Dizziness, Epilepsy, Fear, Headache, Immune system, Insomnia, Learning difficulties, Migraine, Multiple Sclerosis, Multiple personality syndrome, Nervous system disorders, Neurosis, Paralysis, Parkinson's Disease, Psychosis, Righteye problem, Schizophrenia, Senile

Dementia,
Tiredness,
Tremor,
Vomiting

BROW Allergies,
Amnesia,
Anxiety, Blood circulation to head,
Blindness,
Brain Tumor,
Cataracts,
Cancers,
Chronic tiredness,
Crossed eyes,
Deafness,
Dizziness,
Drugs,
Dyslexia, ENT,
Ear-ache,
Fainting spells,
Glaucoma,
Growth issues,
Headaches,

High blood pressure, Hormonal imbalance, Insomnia, Left eye problem, Long-sight, Migraine, Nervousness, Nervous Breakdowns, Scalp problems Short-sightedness, Sinus Problems, Sty, Tension, Tension Headaches, Tiredness, Tremor, Visual effects, Vomiting

THROAT | Asthma, Bronchitis, Colds,

	Cough, Ear Infections, Fear, Hearing Problems, Hay fever, Hoarseness, Laryngitis, Lost Voice, Mental confusion, Mouth Ulcers, Pain in upper arm, Sore Throat, Stammer, Stiff neck, Teeth/Gums, Thyroid Problem, Tinnitus, Tonsils, Too much talking, Upper digestive track, Vomiting, Whooping cough
HEART	Allergies, Asthma, Blood circulation, Breast Cancer, Bronchitis, Chest

Congestion, Circulation problems, Cough, Fatigue, Heart Diseases, High Blood pressure, Hyperventilation, Immunity, Influenza, Lungs, Nail biting, Pain in lower arms/hands, Pneumonia, Respiratory problem, Shortness of breath, Sleep disorders, Smoking, Tremor

SOLAR — Abdominal cramps, Acidity, Anorexia, Bulimia, Chronic tiredness, Diabetes, Digestive

	problems, Eating disorder, Fear, Food Allergies, Gastritis, Gall bladder problems, Gall stones, Heartburn, Hepatitis, Jaundice, Kidney problems, Less immunity, Liver problem, Pancreatitis, Peptic Ulcer, Smoking, Stomach problems, Shingles, Ulcers, Vomiting
SACRAL	Addiction to junk food, Alcohol, Backache, Bedwetting,

Bladder, Creative Blocks, Cystitis, Fear, Fertility, Fibroid, Miscarriages, Fibroids, Frigidity, Hips, Impotency, Irritable Bowel, Kidney problems, Menstrual Problems, Muscle Spasms, Ovarian Cysts, Over-eating, Pre-menstrual Syndrome, Prostates Disease, Stomach problems, Testicular Disease, Uterine Fibroids, Vomiting, Womb problem

ROOT — Addictions, Addictive Behavior, Ankle problems, Anorexia, Backaches, Blood diseases, Bones, Cold feet, Constipation, Colitis, Depression, Diarrhea, Eczema, Frequent urination, Gambling, Glaucoma, Hemorrhoids, Hips, Hypertension, Impotence, Itching, Kidney stones, Knee problems, Leg cramps, Menstrual Problems, Money addiction, Migraines, Obesity, Pain at base of spine, Piles, Prostate cancer, Rectal cancer, Spine problem, Sciatica, Skin problems, Stomach problems, Swollen Ankle, Weak legs, Weight problems

Chapter 22: Physical Healing

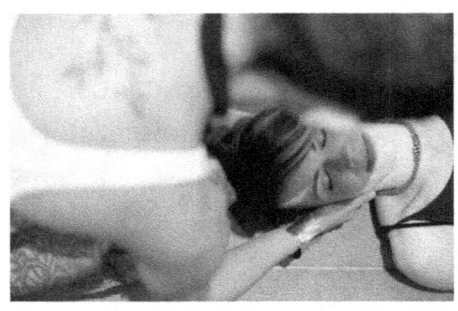

Reiki is a holistic healing practice. That means it can heal the physical body, emotional/mental body, and the spiritual body. When it comes to physical healing, it is easy to think that the body need medicine or massage or physical manipulation to heal physical pain or physical diseases.

This isn't always the case. Imbalances in the body create dis-ease, which then leads to physical pain and even illness and disease. While medication and physical manipulation of the body might offer relief from symptoms, healing has to go straight to the source in order for the healing to truly be effective.

Reiki is not a miracle cure. It is not a heal all method. However, the benefits that Reiki offers sometimes give the body what it needs in order to find its balance, relief, and healing. There are no guarantees, but Reiki is powerful and can accomplish great things in the body.

That being said, Reiki is a wonderful compliment to medical treatments as it can help reduce side effects from medications and therapies, as well as quicken the recovery process. In the cases of terminal illness, Reiki can become a huge asset in easing pain, providing comfort, and aiding in the mental and emotional implications that arise.

For more serious diseases, treatment can be hard and long and painful. Reiki may not be able to completely cure these diseases, but providing comfort and relieving the emotional, physical, and mental stresses makes a drastic difference for the patient.

This is becoming so apparent that many nurses are taking Reiki courses and getting attuned to Reiki so that they can perform it on their patients in hospitals.

Some diseases and physical ailments that can benefit from Reiki include:

Cancer
Heart Disease
Chronic Pain
Infertility
Neurodegenerative Diseases
Crohn's Disease
Fibromyalgia
Surgical Recovery

Cancer

Most people know someone who has been affected by cancer. Whether they've lost someone to cancer, know someone who has survived or is in remission, or have experienced cancer themselves. There are so many kinds of cancers and they are aggressive, usually fast, and can result in a lot of physical and emotional symptoms.

The treatments for cancer are hard. They can sometimes result in more horrible side effects than the disease itself.

Patients who are going through cancer treatments can lose their appetite, be in constant pain, feel depressed, anxious, scared, and sometimes be completely alone.

When the body is fighting for survival or trying to heal itself, it is so important to be in a healthy state of mind with emotions and be in a spiritually healthy place. The body does have an incredible power to heal itself, but if there are imbalances and the emotions and spirit begin to experience symptoms then the body has to work three times as hard and it essentially runs out of gas.

When being treated for cancer, the body can be in so much pain that getting a light, relaxing massage is too much.

Since Reiki can be performed with holding then hands over the body, it offers a pleasant, non-invasive alternative to therapies that require touch.

There are many documented cases where people who were diagnosed with cancer chose to stick to alternative therapies. When being treated with Reiki there are many cases in which patients went into remission with just the healing power of Reiki. This doesn't happen in every case, and Reiki isn't a miracle cure, however, it has been known to happen. Either that or a cancerous tumor might show significant slowing in growth or even reduction in size as a result of Reiki sessions.

More importantly, Reiki can relieve the side effects of cancer treatments like radiation and chemotherapy. Reiki can help stimulate the digestive system and appetite, curb nausea and headaches, and release negative emotions of depression, fear, and anxiety.

Sometimes the body and mind benefit more from a relief of the symptoms than a flat-out cure to an underlying disease.

Some cancer patients went into remission with Reiki sessions and continue to get Reiki as a preventative measure and have been living with no additional signs of cancer for years.

In other situations, the toll of depression on the body from going through cancer treatments is so debilitating that the person may start to deteriorate faster and get sick faster. Relieving the depression with Reiki then allows the body to benefit from the cancer treatments.

It can also be beneficial to the family members of cancer patients who are trying to stay brave and strong, but feel depressed and overwhelmed. Reiki sessions can help relieve their emotional symptoms as they are watching a loved one suffers. You can see there are multiple ways that Reiki can be beneficial to cancer patients and their families.

Heart Disease

When it comes to heart disease, there are several underlying causes. These include blood pressure, cholesterol, lifestyle, and genetics. Reiki can't heal genetics, unfortunately. However, Reiki is known to lower blood pressure and lower cholesterol which contribute to and promote heart health.

Many heart diseases are a result of long-term imbalances in the body or long-term unhealthy habits. While it is best to focus on changing your lifestyle to prevent complications down the road, like sticking to a healthier diet, not smoking, and reducing stress when possible, Reiki is another good preventative.

Because Reiki corrects imbalances in the body, it can become a preventative treatment for diseases and ailments that take a long time to build up. Of course, as with any preventative, adjusting your own habits and lifestyle is going to be beneficial as well. Reiki can start and help maintain the process while you also create shifts in your own life.

Reiki can be used in conjunction with blood pressure and cholesterol medications. Since it can lower blood pressure and cholesterol, getting tested regularly while getting Reiki treatments is recommended so the dosages of medication can be adjusted as needed.

Chronic Pain

Chronic pain refers to any instance of constant physical pain that the body experiences. Chronic pain can be in any part of the body and can manifest in many ways. It might be a stabbing pain, burning pain, or a tingling, needle like pain. Anyone who suffers from chronic pain knows how debilitating it can be.

Furthermore, the western medical system isn't really designed to help people with chronic pain that doesn't fall into a predetermined category. What this means is that if there is no 'obvious' source of pain, doctors have a hard time diagnosing it.

People who suffer from chronic pain might have had an accident or injury that triggered the pain, or might feel it because of the job they work. There are so many causes of chronic pain and so few resolutions if it isn't a cookie cutter, common problem.

Unfortunately, this means that many people who suffer from chronic pain end up on long-term regimens of pain killers and muscle relaxants. These medications can in turn have side effects that can become dangerous and debilitating.

These experiences with medication and no diagnosis can become frustrating and discouraging leading to emotional and mental symptoms as well.

Fortunately, Reiki energy healing, doesn't need a diagnosis or a known cause to help relieve chronic pain. With static hand positions, or performing Reiki hands off, you have the ability to provide clients or yourself with pain relief without aggravating it by moving the body or even touching the body.

Because Reiki is intuitive and corrects the imbalances in the body, it goes exactly where it is needed. In the case of chronic pain, if there was no obvious trigger, like a physical trauma or accident, sometimes it is a result of an imbalance somewhere else.

For example, there have been cases of clients seeking massage therapy for pain in their feet. The pain is so bad they can barely walk. Through the course of treatments, and in working backwards from where the pain is felt, the source of the pain is traced back to a surgical scar on the low back from fourteen years earlier.

Situations like this are common. Surgeries can be traumatic to the body and as a defense mechanism, muscles and connective tissues jam up. After the surgery heals, those tissues and muscles stay condensed. Over time, that defense reaction spreads down the legs and continues to jam up muscle and connective tissue until it manifests as severe pain in the feet.

With Reiki and chronic pain, it is not uncommon to have to work backwards from where the pain manifests to where the pain originates. Doctors don't always have the insight beyond the scope of their specialty to find the true source of chronic pain.

Many people who have suffered from chronic pain for years will start getting Reiki sessions and suddenly not have to take pain killers any more, or get to lower the dose, or even go from heavy prescriptions to just basic Ibuprofen.

Infertility

Infertility is another highly emotional condition that people can encounter.

Women wanting to have children but being unable to do so is such an emotional experience that it can lead to depression, anxiety, reclusively, and a complete lack of self-worth and self-appreciation.

There are many causes for infertility. Sometimes it is something to do with the woman's body and sometimes it has to do with the man's body. Science can help determine if sperm count is low or if there is a potential problem with the uterus or ovaries. Unfortunately, this doesn't always make the situation better or less emotionally painful.

Any woman that has ever experienced infertility yet who wants to be pregnant knows just how horrible it is to get their period every month, a regular reminder that they aren't pregnant. This kind of physical condition has severe emotional and spiritual implications as well.

Reiki energy can vastly improve the emotional mindset and wellbeing of women and men who are struggling with infertility. Just like with cancer, when that emotional and spiritual energy comes back into alignment, the body can focus on healing itself.

More than that, Reiki can help heal imbalances in both men and women so help the production and secretion of fertility hormones and improve their chances of getting pregnant.

There are many accounts of women who had tried everything to get pregnant and were going through fertility treatments with no luck. After receiving Reiki healing sessions, they would suddenly get a viable embryo for the first time in years! It sounds almost like magic, but the truth is, the body is capable of healing itself in many instances. Reiki just points the way.

As with cancer, Reiki isn't a miracle cure for infertility and sometimes can only treat the emotional and spiritual symptoms rather than the core cause, but never underestimate the difference a positive mindset can make.

Neurodegenerative Disease

Dementia, Parkinson's Disease, and Alzheimer's Disease are some of the most well-known neurodegenerative diseases.

There are no cures to these diseases, only treatments.

A neurodegenerative disease occurs in the brain when the brain's ability to communicate with parts of the body begins to deteriorate. As with dementia and Alzheimer's disease, the memory is severely impacted. People lose entire chunks of their lives and their pasts. They can forget family members, spouses, and lifelong friends. More than that they could lose the ability to tie their own shoes because the memory just doesn't exist in their mind anymore.

For neurodegenerative diseases like Parkinson's disease, the brain is no longer capable of communicating with the body and patients begin to lose the function of their body and motor skills.

It is incredibly difficult to watch someone suffer from a neurodegenerative disease and even more difficult to go through it.

Reiki energy healing can actually help slow the degeneration of the neurons and help relieve the physical symptoms of such diseases. There is still a lot to be learned about Reiki and neurodegenerative diseases, but there are documented cases in with Reiki helped to slow the progression of symptoms.

More than that, Reiki provides pain relief for the neurodegenerative diseases that do result in physical pain. Additionally, family members watching someone suffer a neurodegenerative disease can become frustrated, upset, sad, scared, and depressed.

Conclusion

In conclusion it is easy to see why Reiki is picking up such popularity in the main stream now. It is an easy practice to learn and it can help and heal anyone without making them sick from taking medications or painful procedures that can make them end up worse than they were to begin with.

The more you use Reiki the better you will feel about using it. There are three levels of Reiki training and if you feel that you want to live your life by Reiki you can easily find a Reiki Master to take you from a beginner to a Master yourself.

www.ingramcontent.com/pod-product-compliance
Lightning Source LLC
Chambersburg PA
CBHW072003070526
44583CB00015B/1311